T0187332

# THE POWER
# OF HORMONES

# THE POWER OF HORMONES

## The new science of how hormones shape every aspect of our lives

### DR MAX NIEUWDORP

English translation by Alice Tetley-Paul

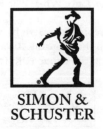

**SIMON &
SCHUSTER**

London · New York · Sydney · Toronto · New Delhi

Originally published by Uitgeverij De Bezige Bij, The Netherlands
First published in Great Britain by Simon & Schuster UK Ltd, 2024

1 3 5 7 9 10 8 6 4 2

Simon & Schuster UK Ltd
1st Floor
222 Gray's Inn Road
London WC1X 8HB

Simon & Schuster: Celebrating 100 Years of Publishing in 2024

www.simonandschuster.co.uk
www.simonandschuster.com.au
www.simonandschuster.co.in

Simon & Schuster Australia, Sydney
Simon & Schuster India, New Delhi

This book was published with the support of the Dutch Foundation for Literature.

A CIP catalogue record for this book is available from the British Library

Hardback ISBN: 978-1-3985-2787-4
Trade Paperback ISBN: 978-1-3985-2788-1
eBook ISBN: 978-1-3985-2789-8

Typeset in Stone Serif by M Rules
Printed and Bound in the UK using 100% Renewable Electricity
at CPI Group (UK) Ltd

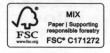

MIX
Paper | Supporting
responsible forestry
FSC® C171272

*For my parents(-in-law):*
*Willemijn, Hannah, Matthias and Leah*

For a list of the various hormones mentioned,
see pages 331–2.

# CONTENTS

# Foreword

*I was (and am) unsure about how I am related to my old self, or to myself from year to year. The hormonal profile of an individual determines much of the manifest personality. If you skew the endocrine system, you lose the pathways to self. When endocrine patterns change, it alters the way you think and feel. One shift in the pattern tends to trip another.*

Hilary Mantel, *Giving Up the Ghost*[1]

This quote from Hilary Mantel about her endocrine disorder endometriosis highlights the extent to which hormonal changes affect people's self-image. It also captures what I love about being a doctor. In the consulting room, you get a glimpse into a patient's life and the way illness affects their character.

I became a doctor because a lot of my relatives worked in the healthcare sector. Although I was more attracted by a career as a diplomat or historian while I was at secondary school, fate (and the Dutch university system) decided otherwise, and I went off to study medicine in Utrecht, like my relatives before me.

Besides a fantastic student life, where I made friends for life and found the love of my life, this course turned out to be a brilliant move. Contrary to my expectations, medicine encompassed so much more than writing prescriptions or performing operations. I learned how to conduct laboratory tests and was inspired when I saw how they helped doctors understand underlying diseases and their associated symptoms – symptoms we then hear about from patients in our consulting rooms.

It was the interactions with patients and the intimacy of the consulting room that led me to study internal medicine at the end of my course. Science played a role too, because there was still so much to be discovered in the field of hormones and gut bacteria. Spurred on by the fact that virtually my entire family suffers from some sort of endocrine disorder – from diabetes to thyroid disorders and even adrenal gland tumours – I decided to specialise in endocrinology, the study of hormones.

After working in this field for almost twenty years – motivated by questions my patients had asked me over the years and to which I didn't always have an answer – I came up with the idea of writing this book. Not only to make the fascinating endocrine system a bit more accessible to anyone who might be interested, but also to put the power of hormones into perspective.

The title of the original edition, *Wij zijn onze hormonen* (literal translation: 'We are our hormones'), refers to the fact that hormones are the conductor of our body's orchestra. It's also a nod to the fantastic book, *We Are Our Brains*, written by my colleague Dick Swaab. While our brain is central to all the decisions and choices we make, hormones, in turn, influence how the brain functions. A hormonal imbalance can play havoc with both our personality and our day-to-day functioning. I recall, for example, a female patient who became sexually disinhibited as a result of an overactive thyroid and ended up in bed with every male patient. It was only when her thyroid was surgically removed that she gradually returned to her old self.

This book was written in the early mornings and late

evenings, because my days were filled with caring for patients, carrying out research and management, as well as meeting the demands of my personal life: a family with young children and a wife who works full-time as a midwife. Despite that, writing proved to be a fantastic source of energy – energy that was badly needed during the COVID-19 pandemic, when I treated people, but also watched them die, on hospital wards.

*The Power of Hormones* is a mix of history and medicine in the broadest sense of the word. I didn't want to write a medical handbook; rather, I tried to confront pseudoscientific claims about the use of hormones as the answer to common complaints. I certainly don't want to suggest that we are slaves to our hormones (or our brains). There is always an interaction between environment, body and mind. Hormones might cloud your ability to make decisions, but they cannot absolve you of responsibility for your own actions.

By writing this book, I have gained an even greater respect for our incredible endocrine system. As doctors, we shouldn't mess with it too much, but we shouldn't become complacent either. We must continue to strive for a deeper understanding of these fascinating bodily substances and keep searching for better treatments. Because, as the famous therapist Salvador Minuchin put it so eloquently: 'Certainty is the enemy of change.'

Amsterdam, August 2022

# Introduction

In 2001, I worked in a rural hospital in Pretoria, South Africa. Pregnant women from the townships – out-of-town suburbs left over from the time of apartheid – would come to the rudimentary maternity hospital in the early stages of labour. Lying on flattened cardboard boxes on the grass outside the building, they would ride out their contractions until the time came to swap the boxes for hard beds hidden behind flimsy curtains inside and delivery could begin. On average, there were about twenty women under my care. Several children would be born each night and I would spend my time dashing between the rooms. One of the children, a girl called Muna, was brought to see me in the outpatient clinic a short while later with stunted growth. She barely responded to attempts to communicate with her and had a puffy face and delayed reflexes. The thyroid hormone in her blood was extremely low, so I decided to give her thyroid hormone tablets immediately to address the deficit.

When I visited the same maternity hospital years later while back in South Africa for a conference, a nurse told me that Muna was severely disabled and cared for at home by her grandmother. Muna's first few months of life without any treatment had taken their toll. She would never be able to live independently and had an increased risk of premature death due to pneumonia or bedsores.

Muna's story shows how important hormones are for our development. We simply cannot do without these substances our bodies make that direct organs and tissues, via the bloodstream, to regulate all sorts of bodily functions. At first, an unborn child is dependent on its mother's hormones. Only after three months in the womb does a foetus develop the cells and organs needed to effectively produce hormones itself. The thyroid is formed in the first trimester of the pregnancy, which illustrates just how crucial this organ is for our existence; indeed, the thyroid hormone is involved in many of our bodily processes.

Due to a dysfunction in the first phase of pregnancy, Muna's thyroid gland failed to develop and she ended up with a congenital deficit of thyroid hormones known as congenital hypothyroidism (CH). In the Netherlands, approximately eighty children are born with this disorder each year. It is not easy to diagnose this condition in newborn babies, and there can be major consequences if it is diagnosed too late, as was the case with Muna. This insight led Hans Galjaard, who was an emeritus professor of human genetics at Erasmus University Rotterdam, to put routine screening for congenital conditions in the Netherlands on the political agenda. Thanks to his efforts, Dutch hospitals and maternity units have been taking blood samples from all newborn babies since 1974 by means of a heelprick test. Partly motivated by the fact that his brother died of a congenital condition at a young age,[1] Galjaard kickstarted these tests, which now screen for thirty-two congenital diseases, after exhaustive political lobbying. As Galjaard put it: 'Better to prevent than not be able to cure.'

As a result, thousands of children have been spared Muna's

fate. I see them in my clinic as lively thirty-somethings, whose lives have been changed for ever thanks to that one thyroid tablet per day (and Galjaard's forward-looking view).

# A brief history of hormones

The term 'hormones' was coined by the British physiologist Ernest Starling and his brother-in-law William Bayliss in 1902. They studied how our digestive system works and how food can be broken down and absorbed by certain substances in the intestine.[2,3]

Two years later, their Russian colleague, Ivan Pavlov, won the Nobel Prize for Physiology or Medicine for his research into the digestive system.[4] Pavlov, chiefly known for his research into conditioning and after whom the acclaimed Pavlovian response is named, used experiments to demonstrate the role of the nervous system in our digestion. But Bayliss and Starling found that digestion also took place in laboratory animals with damaged nervous systems due to the release of special substances into the blood from neighbouring glands. One of these substances was what they called *secretin* (from the verb 'to secrete') – the first of a now extensive group of substances that control our lives in invisible yet far-reaching ways.

It was also Bayliss and Starling who proposed the term *hormone* – Ancient Greek for 'impetus' or 'to set in motion' – as a collective name for these substances. Hormones are signalling molecules created by endocrine (hormone-producing) glands. These molecules travel via the blood and other bodily fluids to their destination – specific cells or organs – where they carry out their work. Most hormones have a central regulatory function; they can either set processes in motion or inhibit them. They also interact with each other.

Our endocrine system's headquarters are found in the centre of the brain, right behind our eye sockets. That's where the hypothalamus and the pituitary gland are located, the size of a strawberry and a pea respectively. Both groups of specialised nerve cells form part of our emotional brain, the limbic system (which you will read more about in Chapter 5). They control both our nervous and our endocrine systems like army generals, keeping a close eye on all the troops.

The effects of these important signalling substances had, however, already been observed fifty years before Starling and Bayliss. In an experiment carried out in 1849, the German scientist Arnold Berthold compared castrated male chickens (capons) with their non-castrated brothers, and found that the first group experienced physical and behavioural changes.[5] For example, the capons were unable to crow. What was striking was that when the testes were restored (by re-implantation or transplantation), and thus the production of the hormone testosterone, the chickens were able to crow again. Similar experiments continue to capture the imagination of writers and scientists to this day, not least because they allude to the existence of an elixir for 'eternal' youth.

The opera *A Dog's Heart* by the composer Alexander Raskatov is a wonderful example of this. Inspired by a novella by Mikhail Bulgakov from 1925,[6] the opera tells the story of the street dog Sharik, who is implanted with the pituitary gland and testicles of a notorious criminal. The animal then turns into Sharikov, a vulgar, destructive human whose behaviour and choices fall prey to his hormone-driven urges. Only a second operation is able to offer salvation to this testosterone-riddled dog ...

References to hormones can be found in older literature too, if we read between the lines – for instance, in the Old Testament. Although techniques to demonstrate the presence of hormones in blood did not exist in those days, their 'momentum' is described: 'the life of flesh is in the blood' (Leviticus 17:11). Certain characters in the Bible probably had congenital hormonal conditions, such as the giant Goliath, who likely had excessive growth hormone. The Egyptian god Bes's dwarfism and Cleopatra's irritability and great energy could also very well have been caused by abnormal thyroid glands.

Let's return to the fascination with the male hormone for eternal youth. In 1889, the 72-year-old Mauritian-French neurologist Charles Brown-Séquard injected himself with testicular extracts from animals to see what would happen.[7]

I have made use, in subcutaneous injections, of a liquid containing a small quantity of water mixed with the three following parts: first, blood of the testicular veins; secondly, semen; and thirdly, juice extracted from a testicle, crushed immediately after it has been taken from a dog or a guinea-pig.

Although the professor was relatively healthy for his age, before he began experimenting on himself he regularly complained of fatigue after a hard day's work, suffering from heartburn and painful joints and muscles. The latter was likely wear and tear as a result of osteoarthritis, which is very common among older people.

In May and June of that year, Brown-Séquard injected himself as many as ten times every day. Almost immediately, the vitality and energy seemed to return to his body; he felt stronger and could run upstairs again. His biceps seemed to increase significantly in circumference, he no longer felt fatigued and he is said to have regained his virility. Testosterone (more about this in the following chapters) is, however, a fat-soluble hormone, and given the fact that Brown-Séquard's injections were water-based, it is perfectly possible that a placebo effect was at play here.[8]

This and other cases have greatly accelerated our understanding of hormones over the past century. Thanks to technological progress, hormones can be extracted from animal material and injected into humans and other animals to observe their effects. This has not only led to many new, important insights for medical science – resulting in several Nobel Prizes between 1920 and 1930 for the discovery of today's best-known hormones oestrogen (female hormone), testosterone (male hormone) and progesterone (which plays an important role in the implantation of the embryo in the lining of the womb) – but it has also had major social, societal and economic effects. The development of the contraceptive pill in the 1950s, for example, had a tremendous impact on the emancipation and empowerment of millions of young women. Successful hormone treatments for numerous conditions have reduced the general burden of disease and simultaneously led to huge opportunities for the pharmaceutical industry.

Unfortunately, our hormone helpers haven't always cut a good figure. Since the publication of Rachel Carson's *Silent Spring* in 1962 – in which the American biologist drew attention to the disastrous impact of agricultural pesticides on the environment, the quality of our food and our own bodies – we have a better understanding of the extent to which these toxins can interfere with our hormonal balance.[9] To cite one unfortunate example: injecting patients with growth hormone taken from the brain glands of human corpses resulted in many of them contracting the infectious and fatal Creutzfeldt-Jakob disease (the human equivalent of mad cow disease).[10] The medication DES, a synthetic oestrogen widely prescribed to pregnant women in the

Netherlands in the 1950s and 1960s to prevent miscarriages, also had major consequences for the health of their daughters, including an increased risk of cancer and infertility; it was found to even potentially lead to abnormalities in their grandsons.[11]

As with Muna, the baby who ended up with intellectual and physical disabilities as a result of defective thyroid hormone production, our health and that of our offspring is highly dependent on the right hormonal balance. In this book, I will explain the influence of the various hormones and the relationship between them throughout the different stages of life – from the cradle to the grave. I will also delve deeper into the consequences of a lack or excess of hormones and the sometimes destructive effect of these powerful endogenous substances on our mental and physical well-being. I hope, like me, you will become fascinated by the wonderful role that hormones play in our bodies and our lives.

# The Power of Hormones

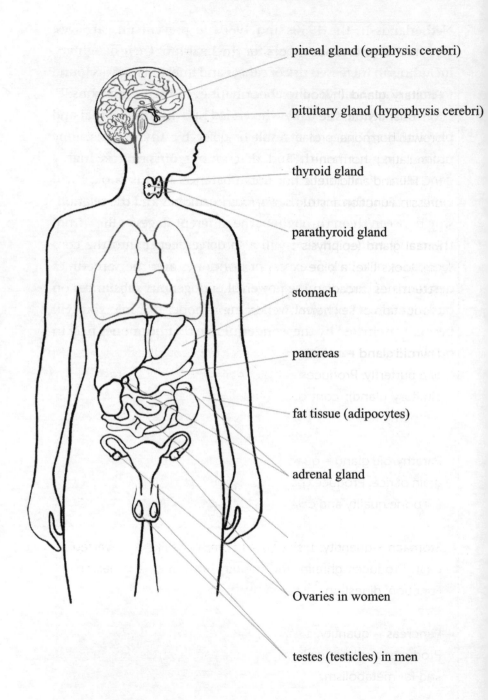

pineal gland (epiphysis cerebri)

pituitary gland (hypophysis cerebri)

thyroid gland

parathyroid gland

stomach

pancreas

fat tissue (adipocytes)

adrenal gland

Ovaries in women

testes (testicles) in men

## Our endocrine glands and their functions

**Pituitary gland** (hypophysis cerebri) – our body's conductor; quantity: 1, size 1 × 1 cm; looks like: a pea. Produces growth hormone, prolactin, luteinising hormone (LH), follicle-stimulating hormone (FSH), adrenocorticotropic hormone (ACTH) and antidiuretic hormone (ADH), also known as vasopressin. Function: instructs other glands to produce hormones.

**Pineal gland** (epiphysis cerebri) – quantity: 1, size 0.5 × 0.5 cm; looks like: a pine cone. Produces melatonin. Function: determines circadian rhythm and sleep quality, inhibits the production of sex hormones until puberty.

**Thyroid gland** – quantity: 2, size 5 × 3 cm; looks like: the wings of a butterfly. Produces T4 and T3 (via TRH and TSH from the pituitary gland); controls metabolism, heart rate and body temperature.

**Parathyroid gland** – quantity: 4, size 0.5 × 0.5 cm; looks like: a grain of rice. Produces parathyroid hormone (PTH), important for bone quality and calcium regulation.

**Stomach** – quantity: 1, size 30 × 10 cm; looks like: an inverted pear. Produces ghrelin (the hunger hormone) and gastrin. Function: digestion.

**Pancreas** – quantity: 1, size 14 × 3 cm; looks like: a flat pear. Produces insulin and glucagon. Function: controls sugar level and fat metabolism.

**Fat tissue** (adipocytes) – present throughout the body, especially abdominal area, size varies; looks like: semolina pudding. Produces leptin and oestradiol (from testosterone). Function: energy supply, elasticity of the skin.

**Adrenal gland** – quantity: 2, size approx. 1 × 1 cm; looks like: a thimble. Produces aldosterone, cortisol, oestrogen, DHEA (dehydroepiandrosterone) and testosterone under the influence of CRH (corticotropin-releasing hormone) from the hypothalamus and ACTH from the pituitary gland. Important for: blood pressure, maintaining sugar and salt levels, immune system and libido. The adrenal medulla produces (nor)adrenaline, important for the stress response.

**Ovaries** in women – quantity: 2, size 5 × 3 cm; look like: almonds. Produce oestrogen, progesterone and testosterone under the influence of GnRH (gonadotropin-releasing hormone), FSH and LH via the pituitary gland. Function: menstrual cycle, breast development, reproduction, bone mass and bone quality.

**Testes** (testicles) in men – quantity: 2, size 4 x 5 cm; look like: eggs. Produce testosterone. Important for: sperm, reproduction, sexual desire, muscle mass, beard growth, bone mass and bone quality.

**Duodenum** – quantity: 1, size 20 x 25 cm; looks like: a bicycle tyre. Produces cholecystokinin (CCK), serotonin, glucagon-like peptide (GLP-1). Function: digestion.

# 1

# First the Egg,
# Then the Chicken

*Pregnancy and Birth*

Today I am seeing Anna, an elegant 35-year-old woman, in my outpatient clinic. Anna and her boyfriend have come for a consultation because she is struggling to get pregnant. She hasn't had a period for two years either, even though she hasn't had a coil for any of that time. Her menstrual cycle was normal during puberty but became irregular when she started her law studies in her late teens. Other doctors such as her gynaecologist haven't found any abnormalities and the psychiatrist ruled out anorexia nervosa as a possible cause. Anna looks slightly embarrassed when she tells me she's a high achiever: a perfectionist, but with low self-image. She often feels inferior to other women and compensates for this by throwing herself into her work. She has been seeing a psychologist for the past year, but doesn't feel this is helping much.

Anna explains that she is under 'some' pressure in her job as a lawyer in Amsterdam's business district. She works twelve-hour days during the week and usually works one full day over the weekend too. It is therefore hardly surprising that she isn't sleeping well – just four to five hours a night. Because she wants to maintain her lean figure and look good, she hits the gym hard five times a week under the guidance of a personal trainer.

My examination doesn't bring up any particular issues, so during a subsequent consultation I unfortunately have to tell her that I don't have an immediate solution to her absent menstruation. However, Anna and her boyfriend haven't been sitting around doing nothing. After searching online, they decided to register with a fertility clinic to have Anna's eggs frozen. This will put them in a better position to plan a potential pregnancy.

In the medical world, we refer to cases like this as 'unexplained infertility', probably caused by the psychosocial stress of our western lifestyle with its high efficiency and pressure to achieve. Unexplained infertility is a source of despair for many couples. If stress is the issue, the simple solution is: eat more (i.e. maintain a normal weight) and relax more (reduce stress).

Much has been written about this subject online and this phenomenon has been known about in the animal world for some time. Female mammals that play a subordinate role within the group may fail to ovulate.[1] Research has shown that the status of a female mammal and the resulting stress experienced significantly affects her fertility. High-ranking female chimpanzees not only have more infants, but those infants also have a better chance of survival, probably as a result of better access to good nutrition.

The American primatologist Sarah Blaffer Hrdy studied langur monkeys in the north-west of India.[2] In temple gardens, people serve this species the most delicious meals. Compared with their counterparts in the Indian jungle, these privileged langurs have twice as many young, a surprising number of which are twins.[3] Having offspring is a costly exercise that requires a lot of energy, so nature will only permit this if enough food is available over a sustained period of time. It's as if the species has 'learned' when it is safe to have twins – a subconscious process.

Less is known about how this process works in humans, but we do know, for example, that more girls than boys are born after a period of high mortality in women. The cause of this imbalance between the sexes is unclear, but environmental factors likely play a role. It has been known for a long time in the field of economic sciences, for example, that relatively more male babies are born during a war, probably to restore the balance between the sexes.[4] In short, the interplay between environment, nutrition, psychosocial stress and the functioning of our reproductive organs is complex. And although I wouldn't like to compare Anna to a chimpanzee, her story also shows that our physical and mental health are closely intertwined – a good starting point to demonstrate how our hormones work.

In this chapter you will read about the role hormones play in pregnancy and birth: in the development of egg and sperm cells, in getting pregnant, in the baby's sex and the mother's immune system, and in both the physical and mental well-being of the mother during and after childbirth. And finally, about hormonal changes in expectant fathers.

## Hormones, reproduction and environment

Hormones play a key role in the creation of new life. This is probably the single most important function hormones have in our existence; there is no new life without hormones. They work together meticulously – and miraculously – in a complex network of substances that stimulate and inhibit each other. By doing so, they not only ensure that egg and sperm cells are created, but also that the meeting between the egg and sperm happens at the right place and the right time. This process doesn't only take place low down in the abdomen. The endocrine system controls our body from deep within our brain – much like a mobile network with several transmission masts.

Reproduction therefore starts in your brain; the pituitary gland and the hypothalamus are the control centres of your endocrine system (as well as your nervous system). From puberty onwards, the hypothalamus in men *and* women produces GnRH (gonadotropin-releasing hormone).[5] This causes the other endocrine gland, the pituitary gland, to produce FSH (follicle-stimulating hormone) and LH (luteinising hormone). LH triggers ovulation and enables a fertilised egg to implant in the uterus. Both hormones enter your bloodstream, after which they travel to your gonads (testes or ovaries). Here, they stimulate the production of sex hormones that help make reproduction possible.

How does this work in men? Stimulated by the LH in the passing blood, Leydig cells, which produce testosterone as well as smaller amounts of the female hormone oestradiol (a variant of oestrogen), are present in the final destination: the testicles. The testicles also contain Sertoli cells that in turn, stimulated by all that testosterone, facilitate the maturation of the sperm cells over a seventy-day period and regulate the production of testosterone via the hormone inhibin B.

Around 5 millilitres of semen (about a teaspoonful) is released with each ejaculation, containing sperm cells that can survive for an average of two days in a female body. The less fortunate sperm cells that are not released during an ejaculation are stored in the epididymis and broken down again after about a month. This process starts in puberty and continues until the end of life.

That's why men can still produce children later in life. This ties in nicely with the biological objective of male reproduction in nature: to impregnate as many fertile women as possible without being selective about it. However, see the boxed section 'Sperm crisis?' as to why there are downsides to this.

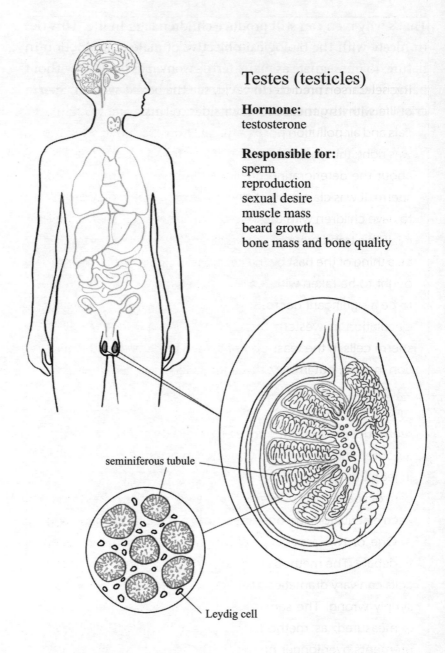

## Testes (testicles)

**Hormone:**
testosterone

**Responsible for:**
sperm
reproduction
sexual desire
muscle mass
beard growth
bone mass and bone quality

seminiferous tubule

Leydig cell

## Sperm crisis?

Rachel Carson predicted it back in the 1960s: our western way of life with its genetically modified food, exposure to chemicals and air pollution poses a threat to our existence.[6] And she was right: thirty years later, the first alarming reports followed about the deteriorating quality and declining production of sperm. It was claimed that one in five men would only be able to have children with the help of IVF due to poor sperm quality. If this trend were to continue, (male) reproduction would be a thing of the past by the year 2110.[7] Although this assertion ought to be taken with a pinch of salt, there certainly seems to be a significant decrease in the number of sperm cells per ejaculation in western men. There were around 47 million sperm cells in the teaspoon of semen produced per ejaculation in 2010, but in 1973 this figure was twice as high (almost 99 million sperm cells).[8] Sperm motility is also decreasing,[9] meaning there are ever-fewer sperm cells to get the job of reproduction done, and those sperm cells that remain are of a poorer quality, too. The concept of 'strength in numbers' is in jeopardy here, as it has long been known that only 0.1 per cent of sperm cells ultimately reach the fallopian tubes during each ejaculation and only a few dozen actually reach the egg.

One or two aspects of this nightmare scenario are open to debate. The methods of determining the number of sperm cells can vary dramatically, so it's possible that the figures are simply wrong. The same applies to the way sperm motility is measured; as methods are constantly improving, measurements over longer periods of time are not always directly comparable.

However, the fact remains that the man and his sperm are a weak link when it comes to human reproduction. Being overweight forms a risk factor; because testosterone in body fat is converted into oestrogen, the modern man is effectively depriving himself of his own fertility.[10] The same applies to having children later in life. Although sperm cells are contin- ually in production (unlike eggs, which are all already present when a baby girl is born), they suffer more from environ- mental factors over the course of a man's life; environmental pollution, exposure to chemicals, radiation and plasticisers cause the quality and quantity of sperm cells to drastically decrease.[11] As a result, the man not only becomes less fertile over time, but his children are also more likely to have autistic behavioural traits.

In short: there's no smoke without fire. That's why such reports must be investigated in order to prevent a potential sperm crisis. If you are a man who wishes to have children, don't wait too long and make sure you maintain a healthy weight.

The twelfth-century Mongolian ruler Genghis Khan took this strategy rather literally. In the sixty-five years of his life, along- side his apparently happy marriage that resulted in four sons, he had various other sexual relations that genetic Y-chromosome data suggests has led to as many as 16 million descendants living today.[12] How was that possible? The rape of conquered women has throughout history been seen as a customary reward for soldiers, and the general (Genghis) had first pick.

For women too, the sex organs – the ovaries – are the last stop in the reproductive process. As girls approach puberty around the age of ten, the pituitary gland starts making FSH, which does what it says on the tin: it stimulates follicles. In the ovaries, follicles – sacs containing immature eggs – start to grow that will subsequently produce oestrogen and also progesterone, which helps the egg implant in the uterus.

The big difference compared with the development of sperm cells is the timing. Eggs, though immature, are produced before birth, when a female foetus is still in its mother's uterus. An embryo has several million. For unknown reasons, most of them disappear before a baby girl is born. At the time of birth, there are still around 1–2 million left. It's only around the time that a female starts menstruating, thirteen or so years later, that they are actually 'used'. By that time, there are around five hundred thousand left. Every time a woman ovulates, a couple of thousand die. That's why it comes as no surprise that women are most fertile before they reach the age of thirty and that, as with men, the chance of reproduction decreases with age. Reproduction is possible while stocks last; once they are depleted, menopause begins (see Chapter 8).

## Fertility and environmental factors

While a man's stock of sperm is continually replenished, that's not the case with eggs. This means that harmful external influences, both while a female is still in her mother's belly as well as during her first twenty years of life, only come to light in the event of a pregnancy. And because that egg also contains 50 per cent of the genetic material of subsequent generations, the result of these influences can extend over many generations.

This claim was first made by Professor David Barker from the University of Southampton, who died in 2013.[13] In the 1960s, he worked as a doctor of tropical medicine in Uganda, where he treated many undernourished women and their children. He developed the hypothesis that external factors such as malnutrition and chronic stress during pregnancy can have long-term effects on children. There was no proof of this until a group of Dutch researchers realised that the Netherlands had been in a similarly terrible situation in the 'hunger winter' of 1944–45, and they were thus able to prove Barker's hypothesis. The women who were pregnant in that last year of the German occupation were chronically undernourished. Almost all of their children had a low birth weight.

Led by Professor Tessa Roseboom, the researchers delved into the archives of hospitals in the Amsterdam region. They collected the details of children born in the winter of 1944–45 and called them up for further investigation. Strikingly, it was found that these women and men were, on average, less fertile and more likely to be overweight and have cardiovascular disease. Their hormone balance was also disrupted. Remarkably, their children and grandchildren were also more likely to be overweight and to suffer from diabetes and cardiovascular disease, even though they had been born twenty and sixty years respectively after the Dutch 'hunger winter' – and in better circumstances.[14]

Fortunately, famines no longer affect much of the world and we in the West live in our version of the biblical paradise. There is so much food that almost one in three adults in the Netherlands is overweight. In the United States, this figure is expected to reach almost one in two by 2030.[15] Twice as many pregnant women are overweight or suffer from diabetes, compared with fifty years ago. It's not hard to see how this abundance can have a harmful effect on our fertility and disrupt our sex hormones.

A similar effect can be observed in mice. When the mother mouse follows a so-called 'cafeteria diet' of unhealthy and unbalanced food, and is subjected to chronic stress, this leads to an increased risk of diabetes, cardiovascular disease and reduced fertility levels in her offspring generations later.[16,17,18]

How relevant is this animal research for humans? There are certainly clear indications that environmental factors not only affect our own reproduction and life expectancy, but also that of our (grand)children. All sorts of internal and external forces are at work when it comes to getting pregnant and giving birth to a healthy child. There is such a complex interplay between various factors that it is hardly surprising that for many couples – think of Anna with her chronic stress – things don't always go according to plan.

---

### The menstrual cycle: how does it work again?

A woman's cycle consists of two phases, each lasting approximately two weeks (see also the illustration on page 201).

*Phase 1: from menstruation to ovulation*
FSH stimulates the ovary to grow a few follicles. These fluid-filled sacs that contain an immature egg release oestrogen. In response, the uterus prepares itself for a pregnancy: the mucous membrane becomes thicker with nutrients and other essentials for the implantation of the egg. Oestrogen also signals to the pituitary gland to make more LH. This sudden surge of LH appoints a winner of the follicle contest. This winning follicle can supply the egg for fertilisation.

*Phase 2: from ovulation to menstruation*
The sac bursts, the egg is released and is transported to the uterus via the fallopian tube. A cyst (or corpus luteum) forms

---

at the site of the sac and produces progesterone that maintains the 'warm nest'. If the egg is fertilised by a sperm cell, it implants itself in the uterine wall. If the egg doesn't meet a sperm cell, the cyst breaks down, hormone levels drop and the uterus sheds its mucous membrane: in other words, menstruation occurs.

# Getting pregnant

During her fertile years, a woman releases an egg on average once every twenty-eight days. This egg develops in a protected environment in the ovary before setting off on its journey to the fallopian tube. Here, it waits for a sperm while slowly making its way towards the uterus. If the egg is fertilised, the newly formed embryo can implant itself in the uterine wall.

If the egg and sperm merge, they produce the pregnancy hormone hCG: human chorionic gonadotropin. This is the hormone that makes a pregnancy test positive and it also has the important task of keeping the corpus luteum alive. This is crucial because this corpus luteum (made from the sac from which the egg was released) is the main producer of the hormone progesterone in the first weeks of the pregnancy.

Progesterone has two important jobs to do: it is responsible for thickening the womb lining so that the fertilised egg can safely implant itself and grow there, and at the same time, it signals to the pituitary gland to decrease the production of LH and FSH. This is to prevent multiple eggs from maturing.

Let's start with that first job; you notice just how important progesterone is if your body isn't producing enough of it. The morning-after pill works in this way, by inhibiting the production of progesterone to prevent an unwanted pregnancy. A low production of progesterone can be the result of a corpus luteum that hasn't developed properly and is therefore unable to maintain the pregnancy, but it's also seen in women who are suffering from stress or who are underweight or overweight – all known risk factors for a miscarriage. In both situations, the body seems to give priority to the production of other hormones (namely cortisol and oestrogen), meaning there are fewer nutrients left for the production of progesterone. As soon as women with low progesterone levels are given this hormone as a supplement, they have the same chance, or less, of a miscarriage as any other pregnant woman. The first two months are the most critical; after that, the placenta takes over the production of progesterone.

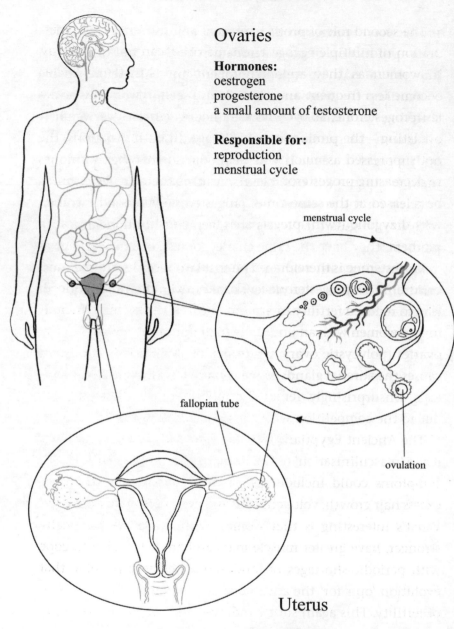

## Ovaries

**Hormones:**
oestrogen
progesterone
a small amount of testosterone

**Responsible for:**
reproduction
menstrual cycle

menstrual cycle

fallopian tube

ovulation

## Uterus

**Hormones:**
pregnancy hormone (hCG)

**Responsible for:**
implantation of the embryo

The second role of progesterone, which is to inhibit the maturation of multiple eggs at the same time, can be seen clearly in women as they approach menopause. Menstrual cycles become less frequent and are lighter, which means you make less progesterone. So even though you are fertile – you are still ovulating – the production of FSH from the pituitary gland is not suppressed as much and the process is less regulated due to decreasing progesterone levels. As a result, multiple eggs can be released at the same time. This is probably also the reason why dizygotic (twin) pregnancies are more common in older mothers.[19]

Progesterone is therefore very important for women who want children. Low progesterone levels, although not always noticed, lead to reduced fertility in around one in seven women, including for women with an unusually high number of follicles in the ovaries (polycystic ovary syndrome, or PCOS). This condition causes the adrenal glands to make more testosterone-like chemicals. Unsurprisingly, female hormones are then less effective due to the competition with the male hormone in the blood.

The Ancient Egyptians were familiar with PCOS, describing it as a 'masculinisation' of the woman.[20] For women with PCOS, symptoms could include decreased or absent menstruation, excess hair growth, voice changes and even personality changes. What's interesting is that women with PCOS are physically stronger, have greater muscle mass and are better able to cope with periodic shortages of food and water; it is possible that evolution 'opts for' the advantage of survival to the detriment of fertility. This again subtly indicates that we do not yet fully understand the hierarchy of hormones in our body, with survival sometimes taking precedence over reproduction.

# Giving nature a helping hand

If getting pregnant the natural way doesn't work due to hormonal or other conditions, synthetic hormonal interventions may offer a solution. Depending on the cause, the egg, the sperm or both can be given a helping hand.

With intra-uterine insemination (IUI), sperm are injected with a syringe directly into the uterus (as opposed to the vagina as with a normal ejaculation), so the first hurdle is already overcome. Knowledge of the hormones helps us out here: the right moment (ovulation) is determined on the basis of the LH surge in the blood. Treatment can also be supported by synthetic hormones at an earlier stage in the process, either by stimulating FSH or injecting it directly. Synthetic hormones are also used in other fertility treatments, such as in-vitro fertilisation (IVF). With this method, sperm and egg cells are taken out of the body and brought together in the lab. If an embryo develops in the test tube, it can be put back into the uterus.

The world's first test-tube baby was Louise Brown from England. Her parents had tried to conceive for nine years with no luck, before Louise was finally born via IVF in 1978. This method was discovered by the British scientist Robert Edwards, who went on to win the Nobel Prize for his work. At first, he was reviled by his colleagues and dismissed at conferences as an unethical doctor. When several hospitals started applying this technique and the children appeared to develop normally, cynicism soon made way for enthusiasm.

The technical feats of this process are astonishing, but they only work if hormones are used in the right way. With IVF or IUI treatment, you start by taking the contraceptive pill to suppress your cycle so that the time of ovulation can be better controlled. Then you have FSH injections that are similar to the signals your own body makes in order to encourage eggs to mature. During ovulation, egg cells are then retrieved from the ovary by means of a needle guided by ultrasound.

As hormones are powerful messengers, this type of procedure does not come without risk. In addition to various side effects such as nausea, fatigue and mood changes, your body can also become overloaded with the externally induced flood of hormones. In two in every thousand IVF treatments, ovarian hyperstimulation syndrome (OHSS) occurs.[21] In this rare condition, too many mature follicles are formed – sometimes more than twenty. As a result, the ovaries become enlarged and fluid and proteins can leak into the abdominal cavity, causing stomach pain. In severe cases, this can even lead to organ failure.

In conclusion, getting pregnant is a finely tuned process, whether or not nature is given a helping hand. This may be why we sometimes refer to a new arrival as a little miracle.

## Being pregnant

Whether this little miracle takes the physical form of a boy or a girl is determined the moment the sperm merges with the egg. The sperm 'determines' the sex; if it passes on a Y chromosome in the genetic material, the embryo will grow into a boy. If the fusion provides a second X chromosome, it will be a girl.

Early in the pregnancy, girls and boys have the same genitals. Initially, a foetus has female structures, but the presence of the Y chromosome makes them disappear and male structures grow in their place.[22] The Y chromosome is responsible for the production of substances that form the male genitals. How exactly does that work? The foetus's genitals produce hormones from early on in the pregnancy, including anti-Müllerian hormone (AMH). In the first two months after fertilisation, AMH ensures that the structures that could develop into female reproductive organs (vagina, womb and ovaries) gradually disappear. As a result, testosterone is given free rein and nine months later a boy can be born.

However, that's not all that AMH does; after it gets rid of the female reproductive organs, the AMH level in the male foetus remains high. It seems that this is associated with the development of the brain, which is being formed during this phase. When male mice are genetically manipulated to produce less AMH, for example, they start behaving less aggressively and less dominantly.[23] Of course, behaviour consists of more than a single hormone level, but the involvement of AMH in the development of the brain could, for example, play a role in the increased risk of boys having autism and ADHD. I will go into this in more detail in Chapter 2.

Incidentally, girls also produce AMH, but only after birth. Its role is to inhibit the enthusiastic FSH to ensure that egg cells don't develop before the start of puberty. Women with the aforementioned PCOS,[24] who often have 'male' features in terms of their appearance and behaviour, often exhibit high AMH levels. However, young girls with normal AMH levels sometimes make more male hormone too, in the adrenal glands. This condition is known as congenital adrenal hyperplasia (CAH).[25] A possible example of this, although not officially recognised as such, has fascinated me for some time: a legend about the first female pope, which has served as an inspiration for film and documentary makers.

## 'Masculine' women

When I was at secondary school in the mid-1990s, we went on a school trip to Rome. I can clearly remember standing by a shrine that was over a thousand years old, not far from the Colosseum, at the intersection of Via dei Santi Quattro and Via dei Querceti. With a smile on his face, our guide told us that this shrine, dedicated to Mary, was reputedly the place where the first female pope John VII (also known as Pope Joan) was stoned to death around 855 AD after giving birth to a baby girl on the street. This story was first written down in 1261 by Jean de Mailly in *Chronica universalis Mettensis*, and became more widely known in 1277 when the Dominican Martin Polanus published his chronicle *Chronicon pontificum et imperatorum*.[26]

According to the legend, after Pope Leo IV died in 855, he was succeeded by a talented young member of the clergy who later turned out to be a woman who wore men's clothing. Riding on a white donkey, this new pope, John VII, was on the way from St Peter's Basilica to the Archbasilica of St John Lateran for the papal inauguration procession when she gave birth to a baby girl not far from the Basilica of St Clement. The crowd was so bewildered by the fact their pope was a woman that they stoned mother and daughter on the spot – precisely where the shrine is today.

This incident may or may not have actually happened, but there are two other reasons why we should take this story more seriously, aside from the altar in the Via dei Santi Quattro.[27] Firstly, in Siena Cathedral there is a row of busts of all the popes from the Middle Ages. Until 1600, the bust of John VII stood there too; it was later removed, possibly suggesting that there is more to this story than meets the eye. Secondly, I first heard about the *sedes stercoraria*, or 'excrement chair', from my Latin and Greek teacher in the Archbasilica of St John Lateran. From the Middle Ages onwards, every papal candidate had to sit on this toilet chair during their inauguration and one of the cardinals would put their hand underneath to check they had testicles. If the new pope proved to be a man, the cardinal would announce: *'Testiculos habet et bene pendentes.'* In other words: 'He has testicles and they hang well.' To which the rest of the group of cardinals would declare: *'Habe ova noster papa'* – 'Our pope is virile.' Although this type of chair can no longer be found in the Archbasilica of St John Lateran, examples can be viewed in the Louvre and in the Cabinet of Masks in the Vatican Museum in Rome. That could explain why, after the case of Pope Joan, a thorough physical examination of prospective popes was carried out before they were allowed to take office.

If Pope John or Joan did indeed look like a man, she might have suffered from adrenogenital syndrome, whereby the adrenal glands produce too much testosterone, resulting in a masculinisation of the body. This syndrome causes baby girls to develop ambiguous genitals and male features, such as a beard. This syndrome is present to a less severe extent in 3 per cent of the population.[28] Thanks to the work of the geneticist Hans Galjaard (see Introduction), in the Netherlands this condition can be detected shortly after birth with a heel-prick test, and can be treated with pills that supplement the shortage of hormones produced by the adrenal glands. As a result, the balance between cortisol and testosterone is restored and young girls' bodies can be protected against exposure to large quantities of male hormone.

Although no clear depictions of Pope Joan can be found, there is a painting by Jusepe (also known as José) de Ribera from 1631, in which he eternalised Magdalena Ventura: a Neapolitan woman with a beard, posing together with her husband while breastfeeding her son. It is possible that there were more of these masculine women in years gone by and the story of the first female pope may be less implausible than it sounds.

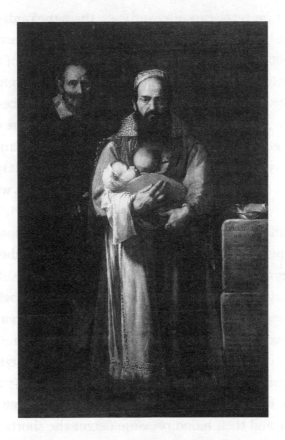

Magdalena Ventura with her husband and son,
painted by Jusepe de Ribera, 1631

## Baby brain

From the thirteenth week of pregnancy, an ultrasound can
determine the sex of a foetus with 95 per cent accuracy. Popular
blogs are full of all sorts of tips on how to guess the child's sex
even earlier than that. What are these based on? That's right:
the effect of our hormones, specifically the pregnancy hormone
hCG. This hormone not only indicates that a sperm and egg
cell have merged and that you are therefore pregnant, but its

concentration level can also indicate the sex. With a female foetus, the hCG levels in the mother's blood are higher; this can be observed as early as the third week of pregnancy.[29]

These higher concentrations of hCG and oestrogen change not only your brain and memory, but also your body. Often, it can take as long as two years to return to your pre-pregnant self. After giving birth, mothers have oestrogen rushing through their bodies for two years and this can influence their behaviour and emotions. Many pregnant women also find they suffer from a distorted sense of taste and suddenly go off their favourite foods. In most cases, this presents itself as an aversion to bitter foods in the first trimester, and a craving for salty and sour foods during the later phases.

What's the point of all this? In all likelihood, an evolutionary adjustment mechanism is at work that instinctively causes mammals to favour products with good (i.e. necessary) nutrients. In general, toxins have a bitter taste and the body actively avoids these during the critical first weeks. Later in the pregnancy, expectant mothers require salt as more blood flows through their body and their blood pressure decreases.

HCG is also responsible for nausea.[30] That sickly feeling doesn't serve a purpose in itself; it's just a side effect of the pregnancy hormone. If the nausea hits you really badly, just remember that the hCG is serving a useful purpose: keeping your progesterone levels high so that more egg cells don't start to mature.

Forgetfulness, a big appetite and strange food-cravings are more commonly seen in women who are pregnant with boys.[31] Why is that? Blame the hormones! Influenced by their higher testosterone levels, these women are more likely to see off a whole bag of sweets or to crave gherkins than women who are pregnant with a girl. This could explain why boys generally have a higher birth weight than girls; they have simply received more nutrients.

Guessing the sex of your child is a fun game for curious parents-to-be. But even before modern medical equipment was invented, people deemed it important to guess the sex in advance – sometimes even before conception. This was not least because in Europe a male heir was considered preferable, in part due to the dowry that parents needed to find for daughters when they married. Centuries before the scientific discovery of hCG and testosterone, French women from sewing and spinning circles realised that a daughter was more likely to cause nausea during pregnancy, while bearing a son was more likely to lead to a bigger appetite. In the fifteenth-century anonymous book *The Distaff Gospels*, six women discuss ancient medical wisdom, including the formation of new life, while spinning.[32] These 'gospels' contain all sorts of interesting tips. Do you want a son? If so, have sexual intercourse in the morning before breakfast, with your husband facing towards the east. How do you know if it worked? According to the spinners, you can tell by the way you walk; if you are expecting a boy, you walk with your right foot first. Still not sure? Get the father to sprinkle some salt over your head while you are sleeping. The sex of the first person you 'accidentally' name on waking will be your future child's sex.

It is not clear how seriously this advice was taken, but distaffs – sticks holding the flax or wool used to make yarn when spinning – feature remarkably often in biblical representations of Sarah and Mary, when the archangels tell them there's a baby on the way.

According to the final myth, women who are expecting a boy become angry and irritable more easily. This brings Voltaire's statement to mind – 'The composition of a tragedy requires testicles' – but has absolutely no basis in science. If you want to win the next guess-the-sex contest, you might as well go along with the expectant mother's hunch.[33] That's because she is instinctively right, without further information, more than 62 per cent of the time. That's a bit better than tossing a coin, but still . . .

In order to bring a pregnancy to term, your body needs to adapt in all sorts of ways. Every trimester has its own requirements. Our hormones play an important role in overseeing all these different physical and mental processes. They ensure, for example, that the nutrients from the food in the mother's intestines reach the foetus. During pregnancy, hormones are therefore both a mother's and child's best friend, making sure that neither go without. An example of this is hPL (human placental lactogen), which temporarily modifies the maternal metabolism. This causes the mother to primarily burn fat for energy, leaving the simple sugars for the child's growth.[34] Female hormones are also known to stimulate the production of skin pigment, an effect that is sometimes also seen with the use of the contraceptive pill (more about the pill in Chapter 7). The increased levels of oestrogen and progesterone can cause irregular brown pigment spots on the face – the 'pregnancy mask'. Fortunately, these pigment spots often disappear after the pregnancy or after stopping taking the pill.

In the final phase of pregnancy, progesterone plays an important role once again by temporarily turning the mother's immune system down a notch. If it failed to do that, the immune system might see the baby (half of which consists of 'foreign' DNA) as a dangerous intruder and want to reject the foetus. So a temporarily impaired maternal immune system is crucial in order to bring the pregnancy safely to term. This can be beneficial for women with autoimmune conditions like rheumatic or thyroid disease, which often become less severe during the pregnancy.[35] However, the flip side of weaker immunity is that pregnant women are often more susceptible to infections and that those infections may then be more severe, as we saw with COVID-19.[36]

# The final hurdle: childbirth

In the third trimester and around the time of birth, hormones once again play a key role. This time, relative newcomers to the hormonal process come to the fore: prolactin and oxytocin. During the later stages of pregnancy, both substances are produced in the pituitary gland, which doubles in size during the pregnancy in order to meet this rising demand for hormones. Prolactin and oxytocin not only ensure that you hold up well during the last months of pregnancy and that you form an emotional bond with your newborn child; they also play an important role in childbirth, influencing when contractions start, when the body needs to recover and when the production of milk begins.

Together with progesterone, prolactin inhibits ovulation, thereby preventing a new pregnancy. The hormone, which owes its name to its role in milk production, primarily provides much-needed mental peace. Prolactin is essential for keeping the mother calm and getting her through those difficult last months. During childbirth, the body increases the concentration of prolactin up to twentyfold in order to speed up delivery and to cement the bond between mother and child in advance.

High levels of prolactin are not only seen around the time of and after childbirth. If your pituitary gland grows for any other reason – for example due to a tumour – large amounts of this hormone can also enter your bloodstream. That was why I once saw a woman in my practice who was 'lactating' despite not being pregnant. It is likely that the first Queen of

England suffered from the same condition. It is reported that Mary I, also known as Bloody Mary, continually believed herself pregnant; her stomach was swollen and she produced milk, but unfortunately no child ever came. She became essentially blind at a young age, likely as a result of a tumour on her pituitary gland.[37]

This is a poignant example of the influence of hormones, and the extent to which they can determine the course of world history. After all, it was in part due to Mary's childlessness that the House of Tudor came to the end of the line and that, after the Stuarts and the Hanoverians, the House of Windsor (formerly called Saxe-Coburg and Gotha) came to the throne and reigned for the past few centuries, right up to the present-day King Charles III.

So women can, even without having been pregnant, produce too much prolactin in their pituitary gland. Medications can also stimulate this process. This may be an unpleasant side effect for some women, but for others it's a blessing, as it means they can breastfeed without having given birth.[38] That's how powerful prolactin's signal can be.

Oxytocin is chiefly released during the first contractions of labour and is responsible after birth for the let-down reflex when the mother hears her baby cry. Oxytocin is sometimes called the 'cuddle hormone'; both men and women produce it after looking at or touching each other for at least half a minute and it's also released whenever you're in contact with your loved ones – your partner, family, friends or children. What's even more intriguing is that socially neglected children with a shortage of oxytocin display behaviours similar to autism; in fact, there is evidence that treatment with oxytocin can make people with autism more sociable.[39] However, because many factors besides oxytocin play a role in the development of autism, more research is needed before this type of oxytocin treatment can be started.

To return to the uterus: thanks to oxytocin, it certainly appears possible to form an emotional bond with the child in your belly. However, it's not just the mother's hormones that set everything in motion. After twelve weeks in the womb, the foetus starts producing hormones of its own, which may even influence when exactly delivery takes place. Research carried out forty years ago by neuroscientist Dick Swaab and gynaecologist Kees Boer indicated this.[40] The Dutch researchers investigated babies 'without brains' (anencephaly) and were able to demonstrate that when the foetus's hypothalamus and pituitary gland are inadequately constructed, delivery happens earlier and more quickly than with healthy children. By releasing hormones, a foetus can therefore determine when the mother's contractions begin, thereby dictating the time of his or her birth. Unfortunately, we don't yet know exactly how this delicate interplay between hormone production in mother and child works. We do know, however, that certain hormones can be used as a therapeutic tool. That's why a dose of synthetic oxytocin can be enough to bring on contractions in a labour that is failing to progess.[41]

## Pain relief for physical stress

Towards the end of the pregnancy, things become especially difficult for the woman. The child has grown to the size of a watermelon. This is quite an assault on all the woman's abdominal muscles and ligaments, which need to stretch considerably. Fortunately, female hormones help reduce the sensation of pain during pregnancy and childbirth. Patients with chronic pain also often experience a reduction in their complaints during pregnancy, though the reason for this could be that they don't have a monthly oestrogen dip as they usually do as part of their menstrual cycle.[42] During delivery, when the body is under a considerable amount of stress, mothers produce endorphins. These are endogenous morphine-like molecules that originate from the hypothalamus and provide additional, temporary pain relief. Endorphins are perhaps best-known from the field of endurance sport, in particular from the runner's high that is experienced due to the production of these hormones while exercising, which explains the addictive effect of running marathons.[43]

### Endorphins and exorphins: painkillers and happy hormones

The term 'endorphin' is a portmanteau of 'endogenous' (internal) and 'morphine'. Morphine refers to the active substance named after the Greek god of dreams, Morpheus. If you have ever experienced the effect of synthetic morphine, you will know why. Synthetic morphine is obtained from the opium poppy, also known as *papaver somniferum* (*somniferum* means 'sleep-bringing'). The effects of morphine have been known for centuries. In the Ebers Papyrus, one of the oldest surviving medical documents (1550 BC), it was recommended as a treatment for babies with colic.[44]

Besides childbirth and endurance sports, substances in our diet (such as fats and sugars) can also release endorphins. Take chocolate, for example: this contains substances that make us want to eat more of it.[45] Gut bacteria can also supply us with additional endorphins.[46] (You can find out more about this in Chapter 6.)

While the body's own happy hormones are released into our brain and bloodstream in a controlled, carefully timed manner, we also have external control over the quantity of endorphins we are exposed to. Biologists suspect, for example, that the natural function of cows' milk is to keep calves close to their mothers, so they keep coming back to drink. If you make cheese from this milk, it contains a lot of casein. This is an animal protein with a highly addictive effect and may explain why people who have long outgrown the nursing stage get the same 'fix' from their weekly pizza.[47]

## Helpful hormones for mental stress

Hormones don't only offer a helping hand during intense physical exertion such as endurance sports or childbirth, but also when people are experiencing mental stress. A pregnancy – with a labour that easily exceeds a marathon in terms of duration – also has a considerable emotional impact. The father of modern medicine, Hippocrates of Kos, was the first to use the term *hysteria*, which means 'womb' in Greek. He used it to describe a situation he considered remarkable, in which more blood travels to the uterus than the brain, resulting in panic and nervousness. The medical term we still use today for the surgical removal of the womb, 'hysterectomy' (literally: removal of the hysteria), also derives from this.

At that time, hysteria or psychological arousal was partly explained by a toxic accumulation of the female reproductive bodily fluids, because it was most commonly seen in widows unable to release those fluids through sex.[48] Until the twentieth century, the treatment of hysterical patients therefore consisted of generating an orgasm, euphemistically described as a 'pelvic massage'.[49] We now understand why this seemed effective; the sudden release of the hormone oxytocin after an orgasm reduces psychological stress and unrest.[50] We also know that a higher level of sex hormones in the blood makes the skin look healthier, younger and more radiant.

During pregnancy, most women feel more emotional than usual. A hormonal explanation for this is the high level of oestrogen over a sustained period of time. The implanted embryo also produces chemicals such as serotonin from tryptophan during the pregnancy,[51] which are likewise closely interlinked with the mother's mental well-being.[52] A dip in these levels after delivery may also explain the infamous 'baby blues'.[53] The body usually redresses the balance within two weeks. However, if the feeling persists, milder mental distress can turn into postpartum depression, which is also associated with lower oestrogen levels in the blood.

Does this mean that depression of this kind can also be cured with hormone therapy? Unfortunately, we don't yet have an answer to that question; we will have to await the findings of ongoing investigations into oestrogen treatment for postpartum depression.[54]

## Hormonal fathers: we are 'pregnant' too

It is not only the pregnant woman who is influenced by hormones. The expectant father also undergoes a hormonal adjustment, with his testosterone levels falling in the last trimester of his partner's pregnancy and experiencing an extra dip after the birth.[55] This does not mean that as a man you suddenly lose your 'masculinity'; instead, you adapt biologically to take care of your child. Testosterone can exacerbate physical aggression and increase libido, traits we would rather not see in new fathers.

Recent research has shown that the labour or 'cuddle' hormone oxytocin can stimulate certain emotions in men. In a US study, thirty young fathers were administered synthetic oxytocin via a nasal spray.[56] The result? When they were then shown photos of their children, the parts of the brain involved in empathy and emotion showed more activity. By contrast, childless men have less oxytocin and more testosterone in their blood; their brains are also quicker to react to sexual stimuli.[57]

Hormones influence behaviour, but interestingly, behaviour also influences hormones. The more time a young father spends with his child, the more his testosterone levels fall, making him less quick to react to sexual stimuli and less likely to act aggressively.[58] However, the hormone balance is restored long before your child takes their first steps.

Apart from more oxytocin and less testosterone, fathers also experience other hormonal changes: increased prolactin levels and decreased oestradiol levels.[59] To start with prolactin: as mentioned earlier, in women this substance inhibits the hormones associated with a potential new fertilisation. The expectant father and his changed male body seem to agree that one offspring at a time is enough. And in the same way that prolactin gives mental peace to women, it also ensures men form a good bond with their child and respond calmly to the sound of a crying baby – also rather important.

It may seem surprising that a man's oestradiol levels drop, but it isn't. Oestradiol is a variant of oestrogen, which is present in a tiny amount in men's blood. It is produced in fat tissue and 'feminises' the brain. A dependent baby benefits more from a caring teddy bear as a father than a hunting-mad grizzly bear, so once again, hormones outsmart the 'caveman'.

Besides hormonal changes, something else sometimes seems to happen in the man's body. It is still unclear whether or not female hormones in a pregnant body are able to change the expectant father's behaviour, but couvade syndrome suggests this might be possible.[60] The word 'couvade' comes from the French 'couvée', meaning 'to hatch' or 'to brood'; in English we sometimes refer to this as sympathetic pregnancy. This is when a man experiences pregnancy symptoms such as nausea, food cravings and mood changes along with his pregnant partner. A striking number of men who are susceptible to sympathetic pregnancy also gain weight during those nine months, especially if the expectant mother is pregnant with a girl.[61] This is a rather nice biological adaptation, as all parties can benefit from some extra energy to see them through those sleepless nights ahead.

Incidentally, couvade syndrome is not a new phenomenon. It was first described in ancient Alexandria by the Greek poet Apollonius of Rhodes (295 BC) who reported how men would routinely go and lie in bed beside their wives in the foetal position during labour to handle contractions 'together'.[62] In some tribes, separate huts were built so the man could find peace himself instead of supporting his wife. In these cultures, this phenomenon was approached from a spiritual point of view, and it was seen as birth by the father.

How does sympathetic pregnancy work? This is where pheromones come to the fore.[63] Pheromones are substances made from our sweat, saliva, urine and faeces that spread between people through the air and by touch, passing signals on to our brains.[64] The receptor for these pheromones is – not entirely surprisingly – found in our nose. During my studies for my US medical exams, I first learned about the vomeronasal organ, also known as Jacobson's organ. This organ in the nasal septum is directly connected with the hypothalamus via nerve pathways. As a result, the body is able to subconsciously detect pheromones, as well as the direction from which they are released (see the figure on page 106).[65] Although scientists long thought that the vomeronasal organ had gradually disappeared, it is in fact still present in almost a quarter of all adults.[66]

A possible explanation for sympathetic pregnancy could be that the pheromones released by the pregnant woman cause the man and woman to hormonally 'synchronise'.[67] This effect is frequently observed. Female lap dancers, for example, often receive bigger tips when they are secreting the pheromone estratetraenol, especially around the time of ovulation when their oestrogen levels are high.[68] The opposite is also true: the pheromone androstadienone found in men's sweat may create a sexual attraction response in women. In short, if you have just become a father for the first time, and you are feeling lethargic and suffering from mood changes, pheromones and the vomeronasal organ may be to blame.

For thousands of years, reproductive hormones have therefore had a huge impact on general physical and emotional health – and not just for women. The fact that men can also quickly adapt hormonally in this way may suggest that the division of male and female social roles in the young family is less black-and-white than it might seem – everything our hormones do is to ensure the survival of the species.[69] Without well-coordinated endocrine systems, our reproduction could be seriously jeopardised.

However, this doesn't mean that every new father is hormonally driven to fixate on the family. Men may also have a tendency for infidelity after having children: the so-called Coolidge effect.[70] This could also be an evolutionary relic, since infidelity causes genes to be mixed and spread more widely, thereby increasing the chances of survival for the offspring. This behaviour, which can be traced back to primitive instincts, can be observed in other species too; for example, cocks are more likely to exhibit sexual behaviour with new hens than familiar ones.[71] Here too, there is a clear link between hormones, brain and behaviour. Without going into too much detail: cheating causes dopamine to be released; this substance activates the oldest part of the brain, where the primitive instinct is found.[72] That's why there is a thick, rational layer of cerebral cortex over this part of the brain, which goes some way to deterring men from philandering macho behaviour when their partners have recently given birth.

To sum up: everyone has a marvellous, self-governing hormonal programme that is continually occupied with enabling the body to function properly. Hormones also help with all sorts of challenges in life, starting with conception, pregnancy and delivery – processes that just wouldn't be possible without this hormonal fine-tuning.

However, to paraphrase the Dutch footballer Johan Cruyff, every evolutionary advantage also has its disadvantage. While our physiology was formed at a time when reproduction was our chief priority, our environment has changed drastically over a short period of time. Our body is essentially equipped for a different environment to the one in which we now need to survive. It does not always correspond with our modern way of life. And that can also lead to problems when trying to get pregnant – for example due to stress, as was the case with my patient Anna.

And even if a person does get pregnant, minor interference during the pregnancy can cause major problems later on, starting with the phase from toddler to teen, as we will discover in the next chapter.

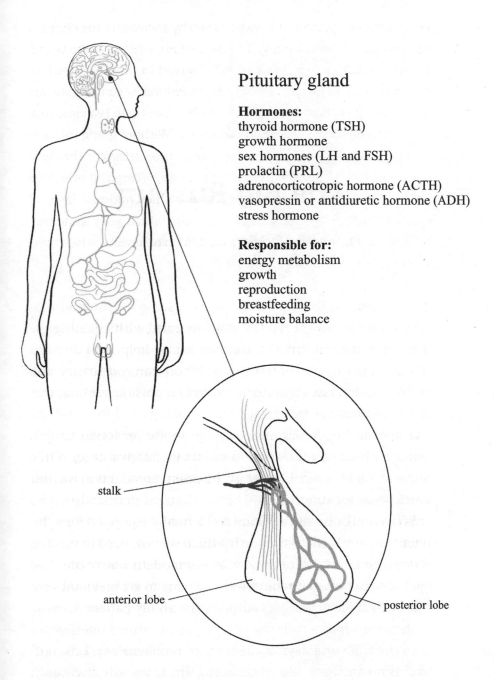

# Pituitary gland

**Hormones:**
thyroid hormone (TSH)
growth hormone
sex hormones (LH and FSH)
prolactin (PRL)
adrenocorticotropic hormone (ACTH)
vasopressin or antidiuretic hormone (ADH)
stress hormone

**Responsible for:**
energy metabolism
growth
reproduction
breastfeeding
moisture balance

stalk

anterior lobe

posterior lobe

# 2

# The Big Run-up

*Pubescent Toddlers and Pre-schoolers*

I wake up on New Year's Eve 2010 in high spirits. It's been a good year, my wife and I are happy, our third child is on the way and I've just started training to become an endocrinologist in Amsterdam. Life seems to be treating us well. I go over to our two-year-old son, who's lying in bed looking as white as a sheet and murmuring, 'Ow, tummy, ow.' Over the past few months, he hasn't been eating as well as usual and he's woken up a few times at night soaked in sweat, but that hadn't given us too much cause for concern.

When I lift him out of bed, I feel a hard lump just below the right side of his ribcage. At first I think I'm imagining it – I've never seen or felt that lump before – but eight hours later our life has been turned upside down. The diagnosis: childhood liver cancer with metastases. It is unlikely he will live to see the end of the next year.

In the following days, a line from Franz Schubert's 'Erlkönig' haunts my thoughts like an earworm. The musical work is based on Goethe's poem from 1782, in which a father carries his ailing child home, riding all night on horseback. Meanwhile, the son, whose condition is rapidly deteriorating, deliriously mumbles that the king of the fairies wants to take him away to the underworld: 'My father, my father, he has seized me! *Erlkönig* is harming me!'

The months that follow are incredibly stressful for our whole family. We stay at Amsterdam University Medical Center round the clock and sleep badly every night. Our son has to undergo a liver transplant with part of my own liver; this entails a serious operation for the pair of us in Brussels. Stress hormones surge through our bodies.

Fortunately, things turned out all right for our son, but our youngest daughter was exposed to elevated levels of the stress hormone cortisol in the womb for almost five months. Although we don't know what the long-term effects of this will be, we had many a sleepless night in the first three years of her life because she was constantly hungry and easily overstimulated. Although she's doing much better now, she has to pay special attention to what she eats because she gains weight much more quickly than the rest of our family.

This can likely be attributed to a mechanism called 'epigenetic change'; if you are exposed to the stress hormone cortisol early in life, certain genes are calibrated differently for the rest of your life.[1] Some of our hormones have this powerful effect; although your genes themselves don't change, they do function less effectively, which is detrimental to your health.

The effects of hormonal fluctuations during a pregnancy can have a lasting influence on the child's developing brain and body.[2] Severe chronic stress during pregnancy can cause irreversible damage to the neurological development of foetuses – just think, for example, of children born during wars or other violent conflicts. In such cases, the child's critical development period coincides with the period in which the stress hormones in the mother's blood are elevated.

Since these hormones affect our immune systems and our brains, the effects are reflected in several of our physical and mental behaviours. This can manifest itself in all sorts of ways later in life, such as poor concentration, fear of failure, deficient general functioning and possibly even schizophrenia. In a large-scale Danish population study of 1.3 million babies born between 1973 and 1995, researchers found a link between major stress and intense grief in the first trimester of the pregnancy (such as the death of a loved one or another trauma) and an increase in the number of deformities and premature births.[3]

Another study revealed that emotional stress in healthy pregnant women is also detrimental to the motor and cognitive development of their two-year-old children.[4] Unfortunately we are unable to predict which children will be affected by problems caused by early hormonal fluctuations in the womb. This is an extremely complex matter, but in general, the earlier and more intense this cocktail of signals presents itself, the greater the impact will be. Hormones can therefore influence our futures in ways so impactful that it's like something out of a science fiction film.

In this chapter, you will read more about the far-reaching influence of hormones on young children, in particular in terms of the effects of sex hormones on toddlers' bodies. You will see that young children encounter a hormonal storm in the first four years of their lives and what this can mean both physically (e.g. appearance and fertility) as well as psychosocially (e.g. behaviour). I will also explain what can happen if you are exposed to too many hormones at an early age, whether from your own body or from the outside world – via food, toys or pesticides.

## Mini-puberty and early puberty

In 1977, the American medical physicist Rosalyn Yalow won the Nobel Prize in Physiology or Medicine for developing radioimmunoassay (RIA), a new technique used to measure the quantity of a certain substance in blood.[5] Her research represented a great leap forward for a range of medical fields, including endocrinology. It was suddenly possible to accurately measure the concentrations of hormones in the blood and to detect internal hormonal fluctuations that previous techniques had been unable to perceive.

An important discovery that ensued from this was that at a very young age – from one week after birth to around two years of age – a hormonal partnership is formed between the brain and the sex organs.[6] During this period, the production of hormones such as testosterone and oestradiol is initiated – a surprising discovery of a phenomenon previously only known to happen during puberty. What is even more striking is the extent of this activity. Although a baby boy's testicles are twenty-four times smaller than those of an adult man, the hormones they produce can rise to levels as high as those in adulthood. For baby girls, the growth of follicles in the ovaries leads to a rush of oestradiol into the blood – and this hormone surge is comparable with the levels adult women experience during ovulation.

This 'hormone surge' is, by nature, different in boys and girls. In boys, the male hormones increase steadily until they peak at around six months. They then take about the same time again to fall to the characteristic low levels. With girls, we see a cyclical pattern in the production of hormones, comparable to that later seen during the menstrual cycle. Female hormones regularly peak in baby girls between their first week of life (when their mother's hormones present in their blood significantly decrease) and their second birthday. The highest oestrogen levels are observed in girls around six months of age – in some cases, these levels remain raised until the start of toddlerhood.

How can this be explained? Almost fifty years after the discovery, we still know relatively little about why this hormonal circus in newborns takes place. The production of sex hormones at a very young age mainly seems to act like a test drive; perhaps the body wants to know for certain whether the reproductive system works before it puts energy into other developmental processes. With such high hormone levels, similar to those observed in teenagers, you would expect typical adolescent features. While a baby doesn't suddenly get pubic hair or acne, behavioural issues do sometimes arise around this time. Researchers therefore refer to this period as 'mini puberty': a relatively short period of two years with minimal external changes caused by a hormonal production process similar to regular puberty.[7] It is a healthy development and for most children their internal hormonal peaks go unnoticed, in part because their nervous system and other organs are not yet mature enough for the signals to be measurable.[8]

It's not unusual for baby boys and girls to encounter swelling of one or both breasts shortly after birth. This often goes hand in hand with spotting: the loss of a small amount of blood from the baby girl's uterus.[9] In the last weeks of pregnancy, the mother's prolactin level increases and the placenta contains extremely high concentrations of oestrogen. After birth, the maternal hormones in the baby's blood suddenly drop, which can cause the baby to lose a small amount of blood from her vagina. This is less common in premature babies than full-term babies. The blood loss is harmless, as is the swelling of the breasts. This often disappears within twelve weeks after birth, when the hormonal supply from the mother drops.[10]

Around 15 per cent of girls exhibit breast growth again at a later stage, usually between six and twenty-four months.[11] It is no coincidence that this corresponds with the period of female mini-puberty, when oestrogen levels soar. This excessive mini-puberty is probably caused by external triggers influencing the balance of hormones in the body (a balance has been prepared by maternal oestrogens). In this case, you do see the physical characteristics of puberty, such as breast growth, bleeding and even symptoms of pre-menstrual syndrome (PMS).

It is not clear what causes this hormonal storm to blow over again in most toddlers. The pineal gland may play a role. This endocrine gland is located in the centre of the brain and, in addition to its role in regulating the circadian rhythm, also appears to be involved in suppressing the production of sex hormones until puberty begins.[12] Could it then be the case that the key to our behaviour can be found in the pineal gland?

That's what René Descartes believed. With his statement *'Cogito, ergo sum'* ('I think, therefore I am'), the French philosopher claimed that the body influences our thoughts and vice versa. Four centuries ago, long before the terms hormones and mini-puberty were coined, he came up with the idea that our body's soul is seated in the pineal gland and that this gland controls our mental and physical functioning.[13] Pineal gland or not, Mother Nature always makes exceptions to the rule. One such example is when the sex hormones of young children cannot be restrained and puberty sets in far too early.

The term *pubertas praecox* may sound like a magic spell from Harry Potter, but all it means is 'an acceleration of the onset of puberty'. Contrary to mini-puberty, this early puberty, also

known as precocious puberty, is not harmless. A common definition for medical purposes is the onset of puberty before the age
of eight in girls or nine in boys. For some reason, early puberty
is almost ten times more common in girls than boys.[14] Most of
these patients are six or seven years old, but they are occasion-
ally younger, such as the British girl Hayley Smith, who was born
in 1995. She started suffering from stomach cramps and mood
swings at the age of three and other features of puberty followed
shortly thereafter, such as body odour and greasy hair.[15]

If these symptoms are observed in children at such a young
age, it is important to determine the cause: is it mini-puberty
(harmless) or early puberty (disease), perhaps due to a hormone-
producing tumour? Usually the bone age (to be determined by
X-ray) can provide a definitive answer. This is important because
early puberty has far-reaching consequences. If your growth
spurt starts much sooner, the maturation of cells in your bones
and growth plates (the cartilage part of your bones where they
grow in length) is affected; you often end up much smaller
as an adult, because your total growth period was shorter. In
combination with an increase in weight – by continuing to eat
and exercise normally – this can result in abnormal physical
proportions. Patients like Hayley still struggle to maintain a
healthy weight years later.

In addition to physical effects, early puberty can also have
psychosocial consequences. This can lead to poor performance
at school and an increased likelihood of taking drugs compared
to their healthy peers. Furthermore, these children often struggle with being different from the norm and can feel embarrassed
or lonely.

Fortunately, something can be done about it. In almost
all cases, *pubertas praecox* is treated with the same hormonal
injections that are used to suppress puberty in transgender

children (see Chapter 4). Medicine has therefore found a magic wand with which the body's own production of hormones can be put on pause. Later, when the injections are stopped, the puberty movie automatically continues from where it left off.

## Endocrine disruptors

What triggers the rapid increase in hormone concentrations during mini-puberty or early puberty? Disrupted hormone levels may have an internal cause, as previously mentioned, but they can also be triggered by external factors, such as diet.

A few years ago, Turkish paediatricians issued the following warning: limit the use of fennel tea in very young children.[16] In Turkish culture, fennel tea is a popular herbal remedy for intestinal colic and other digestive issues in babies, due to its relaxing effect on muscle tissue. Dutch mothers are bombarded with the same advice. On the Dutch website Oma weet raad ('Grandma knows best'), it is listed as a child-friendly option under 'Babies with colic'. What is less well-known is that fennel contains anethole, which acts similarly to oestrogen. Too much fennel elevates oestrogen's effect on the body and can therefore lead to breast development, as Turkish researchers found in their study. Fortunately, the noticeable breast growth they observed in the children in the study disappeared again after fennel was taken off the menu.

Besides food products, popular 'natural' skincare products can also promote breast growth in young children. In Australia, for example, an infant developed breasts after the excessive use of body products containing lavender.[17] The internet is full of well-intentioned advice for mothers, but nowhere does it mention that essential oils like lavender can affect hormone levels, even leading to breast growth in boys. You would need to use loads of it, however. These products are healthy, as long as they are used in moderation.

It has long been known that some plants contain hormone-like substances called phytoestrogens, which fall into three categories: isoflavones (such as those found in soya), coumestans (in alfalfa) and lignans (in linseed). In the Old and New Testaments, they are also referred to as 'garden herbs', eaten by people who didn't want to eat meat. The pros and cons of these high-protein meat replacements are still disputed today; I will delve into this in more detail later in this chapter. The long-term daily consumption of these substances can cause the oestrogen level in a young child's blood to significantly increase.

In medical literature, the formation of breasts in young children is linked to soya-based infant formulas, legumes and eating meat.[18] Meat doesn't inherently contain plant-based oestrogens, but it can be contaminated as a result of hormone injections in cattle.[19] Some farmers inject their cattle with hormones in order to increase the yield and to make more profit, but this is bad for the (small) people who consume it; that's why hormone injections in cattle are now banned in the European livestock sector. In the late 1970s, a sudden increase in the use of these substances led to a breast growth epidemic in babies in countries like Puerto Rico and Italy.[20,21] Jars of beef-based baby food were found to contain extremely high levels of the infamous and now illegal substance DES: an oestrogen-like substance that was added to cattle-feed to prevent miscarriages in cows, and which ended up in the human system. Thanks to clear public warnings from doctors and researchers, tighter legislation was promptly passed.

Early breast development is not a thing of the past, however. In some countries (Turkey, Denmark, France and Hungary) we are seeing increasing numbers of young children with breast growth.[22] Some researchers link changes in the appearance of young children with our modern diets: less bread and potatoes, more vegetarian sources of protein and all sorts of cereals. Over the past years, Dutch people have also started eating around 30 per cent more legumes (mainly soya beans) as meat substitutes.[23] Supporters of soya often point to the high life expectancy in Japan and other Asian countries; they view this as irrefutable proof that soya consumption can't do any harm. What's often overlooked is the dosage; relative to body weight, an average Japanese woman consumes considerably less soya per day than a western woman. Soya is also often consumed in a fermented form in Asian countries, such as miso, natto or tempeh, which are different substances in biochemical terms. In the West, we may also be consuming soya on a daily basis without realising it, as it is added to processed products. Think, for example, of vegetarian meat substitutes, but also of the waste from processed soya beans (soya-bean meal), which is one of the most important sources of protein for pigs and poultry. While it remains unclear whether these natural endocrine disruptors can be harmful to our offspring,[24,25] we must be vigilant. Studies have shown that soya products (in infant formula) can affect the development of the child's brain.[26]

At first glance it may seem surprising that we're unable to draw a clear conclusion, but according to researchers such as Theodora Colborn (see page 60), this is partly because the effects of endocrine disruptors are so difficult to investigate. Many years can pass between a body being exposed to a substance and the externally visible consequences of it, and not everyone who is exposed to a substance develops problems. But the fact remains that the endocrine system is still developing in the womb and during the first years of life, meaning that babies and young children are at greatest risk when they or their mothers are exposed to endocrine disruptors.

## The effect of chemicals on our hormones

Theodora Emily 'Theo' Decker Colborn (1927–2014) is regarded as the pioneering researcher of the past century in the field of endocrine disruptors. She was greatly inspired by the work of Rachel Carson and during her doctoral research acquired a vast amount of knowledge in the fields of pharmacy, ecology, zoology and toxicology. In the 1980s, she carried out research into the reproductive and developmental problems of various species of animal.[27] She showed that these animals had been exposed to high concentrations of phytohormones and synthetic substances, such as pesticides, insecticides, soap-like substances and plastic substances like PFAS. Her research demonstrated that these substances can enter the systems of living beings: animals and people. Even low dosages of endocrine disruptors in our environment and in our food can lead to very serious physical disturbances in the long term, such as the effect on sperm quality in men (mentioned previously). Because people are living longer, Colborn claimed, we would see an increase in endocrine and (auto-immune conditions from the 1970s onwards, and recent studies certainly seem to confirm this. (Read more about this in Chapter 7.)

Thanks to the efforts of Colborn and other researchers, the suspected dangers of endocrine disruptors from the environment are now on the agenda of important organisations such as the World Health Organization (WHO) and the European Union. Teams of experts are busy researching the long-term consequences for humans, animals and the ecosystem.

## Plasticisers and pesticides

Endocrine disruptors can be chemical as well as plant-based. Pollutants in plastics, cosmetics, paint and pesticides have been proven to disrupt the hormonal balance. These include the notorious plasticisers,[28] which are used, for example, to ensure that rubber and plastic (such as the teat on a baby's bottle) are supple and flexible.

At the start of the century, German researchers warned of the unhealthy consequences of the 'scoubidou' craze, in which children twist lengths of coloured plastic together to make items like friendship bracelets.[29] Research showed that these strings contained extremely high levels of plasticisers called phthalates, which can enter our bodies via inhalation and through contact with the skin and the mouth. A few centuries ago, the Swiss doctor Paracelsus established that while a substance may not be toxic to touch, it can be so if your body ingests a substantial amount of it. Phthalates are also less powerful than our body's own oestrogens. But we should make no mistake: an accumulation of various endocrine disruptors can have a considerable impact on our bodies. And plasticisers are not only found in plastics.

A 2013 study of girls living in a French industrial area, who were exposed to all sorts of chemical substances, including plasticisers, showed that their oestrogen levels were many times higher than those of girls who lived in a different, healthier environment.[30] The girls living in the industrial area developed breasts at a young age, including a four-month-old baby with breasts of almost adult proportions. There were so many pesticides (DDT) in the barn on her father's farm that she had five times as much oestrogen as normal and had already experienced vaginal bleeding on three occasions. Her father and mother were affected too; they reported a dramatic decrease in libido.[31] Vaginal bleeding and breast development disappear on their own as soon as those external substances leave the scene, but the long-term consequences are currently unknown.[32]

Due to their sensitivity, infants are our metaphorical canaries in the hormonal coal mine. Young children are more susceptible to this type of phenomenon, not only because they have the tendency to explore their plastic-filled environment with their mouths, but also because their liver and kidneys, responsible for detoxification, are not yet fully developed. The fact that babies ingest large quantities of liquids and food, relatively speaking, makes them vulnerable. They also have a relatively high fat mass, fat being a favourite storage place for these endocrine disruptors, which are slowly released from adipose tissue, leading to exposure over a longer time. Based on this knowledge and, above all, the unknown long-term consequences,[33] it's important to beware of harmful plastics until research can provide greater clarity.

## Fertility problems among boys

Balanced sex hormones are also crucial for the healthy development of baby boys. As with girls, deficits or surpluses of both testosterone and oestrogen have major consequences. Boys with undescended testicles have an increased risk of fertility problems, for example. Whereas both testicles usually descend into their proper place in the scrotum about a month prior to birth, in around one in twenty boys one or both testicles remain undescended at birth. This is known as *cryptorchidism*: Greek for 'hidden testicles'.[34] As the testicles are usually located in a predictable place in the abdomen and groin, this is relatively simple to detect and remedy with an operation. It is important that this happens when the infant is still young because testicular cells are especially susceptible to temperature. They thrive in the cooler scrotum outside the body. This maintains the quality of the semen, but also prevents unimpeded growth; in the warmer abdominal cavity, the testicle overheats and there is a higher chance of malignant growth. That's why this medical intervention is usually carried out at a young age – ideally in the first year of life.

---

### People as rarities

Another, much rarer, congenital hormonal abnormality that can occur in very young girls is an excess of their body's own testosterone – in other words, an excessive production not of female but of male hormones. In the eighteenth, nineteenth and even twentieth centuries, these children often ended up as attractions at fairs and in circuses due to their striking physical characteristics, where they were publicly exhibited in popular freak shows. The film *The Greatest Showman* tells the romanticised story of P. T. Barnum, a nineteenth-century American circus owner who owed a large part of his success to people with special hormonal conditions. One of the children who was part of Barnum's collection of rarities at the age of just nine months was the American Annie Jones Elliot.[35] She was born with a strikingly hairy face and body, and was billed as 'The Infant Esau', a Biblical reference to the extremely hairy son of Isaac and Rebecca. Annie already had a distinct moustache when she was just a few months old and a full beard by the age of five. It's possible that she suffered from adrenogenital syndrome (see also the story of the first female pope, on page 32).

---

Other world-famous examples are Julia Pastrana from Mexico and Krao Farini from Laos.[36,37] Their stage names – 'the ape woman' and 'the missing link' (between human and ape) – refer to the presence of exaggerated male features such as excessive facial and body hair. The scientific basis for their symptoms was only discovered years later: they produced huge quantities of testosterone. This is often caused by poorly functioning endocrine organs like the adrenal glands and ovaries.

As knowledge of these conditions increased and the mystery decreased, criticism of these types of exhibits grew. Despite this, a photography project entitled The *LA Circus Congress of Freaks and Exotics*[38] brought performers together as recently as 2007, and the British reality show *The House of Extraordinary People* also captivated viewers in 2019. Circuses aren't needed in this day and age: fearless bearded women like Harnaam Kaur, who owes her facial hair to ovaries that produce too much testosterone, can find fame today via social media on their own terms.[39]

Strangely enough, this procedure barely reduced the likelihood of fertility problems.[40] Something was therefore already awry in those boys' bodies before the operation. The undescended testicles that reduced fertility were clearly the result of an underlying medical condition. After years of scientific detective work, a cause was found: increased exposure to female hormones in the mother's womb adversely affects the quantity of testosterone.[41] Testosterone is responsible for the testicles finding their way to the scrotum, so the shortage of it during pregnancy was what prevented the testicles from descending sufficiently.

Incidentally, the origin of the term testicle comes from an old custom. In Roman times, men would confirm an official promise or oath between themselves by grabbing each other's testicles. It was also customary for men who had to bear witness in a public forum to do so with their right hand on their scrotum as a sign of truthfulness. The term 'testicle' is derived from this ritual: *testiculus* means 'witness' in Latin.[42] If you didn't have any testicles – if you were a man who had been castrated because you had committed adultery, for example – you were unable to testify in court.

This custom is also mentioned in the Old Testament. In the Book of Genesis, Abraham asks his servant Eliezer to put his hand under his thigh to swear an oath. In a more recent example, during the Second World War British spies used existing knowledge about testosterone and testicles to try to subdue Hitler's aggressive character. They knew that Hitler had only one testicle and that he probably produced less testosterone as a result. As part of a secret sabotage plan, the spies discussed the possibility of adding oestrogen to the Führer's meals.[43] As oestrogen supplements have no smell or taste, the food tasters wouldn't notice them. For some reason, this plan never materialised and the British hypothesis couldn't be tested, but considering current scientific knowledge, this experiment could have worked.

How do baby boys incur such an excess of female hormones? As with the baby girls with breasts, through an excess of oestrogenic signals – for example, because the pregnant woman ingests too many phytohormones (plant hormones) through her food. However, less obvious causes such as environmental factors also leave their mark. Pollutants, for example, have been linked to undescended testicles and lower levels of testosterone.[44] A Spanish study showed that testicles were more likely to be undescended in boys living in areas with greater pesticide use.[45] When this type of chemical was subsequently given to pregnant animals, the male offspring were more likely to have undescended testicles and were less likely to be fertile at a later age.

As with the girls, the same applies for the 'bad' plastics: the phthalates. A research study showed that families that lived closest to an acrylic factory in the Hungarian border town of Nyergesújfalu were most likely to have sons with undescended testicles. The far-reaching effect of these plasticisers can also be seen in experimental studies on animals, where 84 per cent of animals exposed to such substances had undescended testicles, compared to none in the control group.[46]

A disturbance to the male hormonal balance prevents the normal descent of the testicles to the scrotum in the foetus. An overheated testicle can't produce enough testosterone, which has major consequences. While male hormone levels soar during mini-puberty in healthy boys, they remain low in boys with cryptorchidism.[47]

The importance of those testicular cells was demonstrated by studies carried out on animals in which descended testicles were actively moved to the abdominal cavity. Within seven weeks, the size of the testicles decreased, as did the production of testosterone.[48] The Leydig cells in particular, responsible for the production of testosterone, struggled to withstand the change in environment and temperature – an undesired development with a long-term effect. After all, testosterone not only ensures that the testicles end up in the scrotum, but it also plays a crucial role in this phase in creating the later sperm cells.[49]

A shortage of testosterone in the first months of life therefore considerably reduces the chances of reproduction. Researchers currently recommend measuring the presence of these important stem cells by performing a biopsy. But if too few are present, all is not lost. The body's own levels can be supplemented with hormone medication, after which the miraculous reproductive system often finds its way to fertility.[50]

## Hormones make the boy and the girl

This simulated mini-puberty, brought about with the help of additional male hormones, can help boys with undescended testicles. In this early stage, testosterone supplements can also be given to boys who don't produce enough of it for other reasons. The supplements increase their fertility as well as the size of their genitalia. These boys usually have underdeveloped genitalia, sometimes to the point where they're barely recognisable.[51] Observant parents of healthy boys may also notice short-term growth of the penis in the first six months due to a natural increase of testosterone.[52,53]

But even if the genital organs have developed as expected, a lack of testosterone can cause the external genitalia to shrink. In that case, the testicles then move slowly towards the abdominal cavity, the scrotum becomes a skin fold and the penis shrinks instead of growing. Treatment with testosterone can restore everything to its 'normal' appearance and function.

For some children, early intervention can prevent a sexual identity crisis in later life. We know that it is relatively common for boys with a 'micropenis' – shorter than 1.9 centimetres in the first months of life – to change assigned gender. A baby born as a boy can quickly become classified as female as a result. Parents and professionals sometimes have to make the drastic decision to remove the micropenis within twenty-four hours of the diagnosis.

Research carried out on a group of these children between

the ages of five and sixteen showed that despite being raised as girls, most of them later identified as men.[54] The fact that these children were exposed to male hormones before birth appears to be the main factor as to why they feel male[55] and pursue interests that are typically thought of as male (more about this in Chapter 4)[56] – irrespective of the sex that was registered at birth.

In exceptional cases, undescended testicles can also lead to serious problems in women. A well-known example of this is the Dutch athlete Foekje Dillema, whose athletic prowess in the early 1950s, especially in sprinting, was possibly due to the fact she had higher levels of testosterone than other women.[57] This caused an uproar and raised questions about her actual sex. As Dillema refused to undergo a medical examination, she received a lifetime ban from the Dutch Athletics Union, who claimed she was 'not a girl'. The dejected athlete didn't protest, and Dillema didn't race again for the rest of her life. She was stripped of her personal record for the 200 metres, and she died in 2007 after living a life away from the spotlight in Friesland.[58] DNA tests later revealed that she was biologically both a man and a woman (also known as genetic mosaicism), as a result of which she reportedly had small undescended testicles in her abdomen.[59]

## Boys vs. girls: Behaviour in play

So far we have mainly discussed the physical aspects of a hormonal imbalance in early childhood. But hormones also have a significant influence on our behaviour through all the phases of life. Just think of the behavioural changes in your average teenager. Most women would also agree that their mood is influenced by their menstrual cycle. So it wouldn't be too far-fetched to assume that the hormonal storm during mini-puberty can also mould the toddler's brain,[60] especially because it takes place during a period of intensive brain development.[61] We sometimes refer to 'the terrible twos' or 'threenagers', but besides difficult, headstrong behaviour, it seems that some stereotypical behaviour can also be attributed to sex hormones and mini-puberty.

I already mentioned that mini-puberty differs between boys and girls in physical terms, but clear differences can also be seen in social terms. An example of such gender-typical behaviour is the way in which girls and boys play, where the connection between gender and a natural preference for certain activities is even more evident.[62] There is no doubt that it is, to a large extent, pre-programmed in our brain, as Dick Swaab explains in his book *We Are Our Brains*,[63] but hormones can certainly play an influential role in how the brain develops during and after birth.

Many parents observe that toddler and pre-school girls generally prefer playing with dolls and toy kitchens, whereas boys are naturally more drawn to aeroplanes and construction kits. Of course, such a preference can't be detached from the child's environment and the toys that are on offer, but the blueprint already seems to be partly ingrained via our hormones. Girls with more male hormones tend to favour toy cars, despite encouragement from their parents to play with 'typically girly toys'.[64] How toddlers play and what they play with is not only related to hormone production at that time, but it can also be determined by hormonal fluctuations they experienced as newborns. A Finnish study demonstrated, for example, that fourteen-month-old boys with higher testosterone levels during mini-puberty showed significantly less interest in dolls, whereas higher levels of testosterone in the girls led to a fascination for toy trains considerably more often.[65]

English researchers took penile growth in the first three months after birth as an indication of early exposure to testosterone in boys and saw a link with more 'boyish behaviours' during toddlerhood, such as rough-and-tumble play and climbing.[66] The timing of these hormonal surges plays a striking role here too. There was no correlation between the growth of the genital organ after the first three months of life and typically boyish interests at a later age.[67] An effect on behaviour and brain therefore seems to be limited to exposure to sex hormones during the first months of life.

Besides play behaviour, the curiosity of young children for their environment also appears to stem from hormonal fluctuations during mini-puberty. The aforementioned anti-Müllerian hormone (AMH, see Chapter 1), produced by the testicles to ensure the male foetus doesn't develop any female sex organs, stimulates curiosity for new environments. Research with rhesus monkeys revealed that male young with higher levels of AMH in their blood were more likely to go off exploring away from the safety of their mothers than their brothers with lower concentrations of this hormone, or their sisters, who naturally have lower levels of AMH in their blood.[68] This can be explained from a biological point of view; in the animal world, males often have to leave the nest to form their own family. Females have a different survival strategy and therefore invest more in mutual interaction with peers.[69] The tendency – in the human world – for boys to wander the streets with friends and girls to sit in their rooms chatting with friends could therefore simply have a hormonal basis. Social conditioning plays a major role too.

# Autism and IQ

An insight into mini-puberty can explain more than innocent preferences like these. It may also help us gain a better understanding of conditions that are more prevalent in boys than girls, such as autism. Autism goes hand in hand with poor social skills and communication disorders: suspected characteristics of an excessive masculinisation of the brain.[70]

There does appear to be a connection between exceptionally high concentrations of testosterone during mini-puberty and scores on autism screening questionnaires. Results from a study carried out in New Zealand found a connection between the level of AMH (and inhibin B, which inhibits the production of sperm cells) and the number of autistic traits in boys.[71] Research into the link between mini-puberty and specific conditions is still in its infancy. Due to the complex interplay of timing and hormone levels, it will take a while before hypotheses can be verified. What we do know is that the early hormonal circus influences the young human body in myriad ways.

Even IQ levels appear to be linked to mini-puberty. Long-term research carried out on boys with undescended testicles shows that a shortage of testosterone at an early age reduces the effectiveness of the genes involved in memory and other cognitive functions.[72,73] This could partly explain why boys who do not go through mini-puberty because their testicles have not descended often perform worse at school. Early oestrogens could therefore form the basis for a flair for languages[74] and communication skills, and androgens (the collective name for male sex hormones) for spatial awareness.[75]

## Mini-puberty offers great opportunities

Considering the influence it has, it is surprising that so little attention is paid to mini-puberty. If you search for 'puberty' in scientific literature, not even 3 per cent of articles deal with the first few months and years of our lives, when our sex hormones surge. This is an oversight, as there is still a huge amount to be investigated and gained in this field. A good hormonal balance in this early phase of life could have an even greater impact on our physical and mental development than during 'real' puberty, when not only the sex organs but also the brain are already formed.

The discovery of the existence of mini-puberty also opened up doors for the detection of serious conditions at a very young age. A shortage of sex hormones in a newborn can, for example, signal a general problem in the pituitary gland. In the past, a defective pituitary gland often went unnoticed, with all sorts of complaints – and sometimes even a fatal outcome – as a result. If doctors can better recognise the signs of a lack of mini-puberty, they can also detect and treat an underperforming pituitary gland more quickly, thereby decreasing the likelihood of illness and death.

As well as its importance for the health of babies and toddlers, a better understanding of mini-puberty could also help treat conditions in adults. Think, for example, of the mysterious, persistent fertility problems following the surgical treatment of boys with undescended testicles. Some (dangerous) endocrine diseases that affect the elderly, caused by the overproduction of hormones, also have a variant that affects babies. A greater insight into the difference between the two variants could generate new treatment methods. To sum up, there are major medical opportunities in store if more scientific attention is paid to mini-puberty.

And what can we, as parents of young children, do in the meantime? Disturbances to the hormonal balance of toddlers and pre-schoolers appear to influence so many aspects of adult life that it's crucial to look critically at diet and environment. Make sure you don't feed your young daughter too many of those plant-based oestrogens and that she doesn't chew on bad plastics too often. And if your baby boy has undescended testicles, ensure that he is operated on as soon as possible after birth.

Things seem to settle down a bit in the years after mini-puberty, at least in terms of hormones. We still don't know a lot about that, so there's not much to say about hormonal fluctuations and the effects of endocrine disruptors in the period from four to ten years of age: the calm before the storm of real puberty.

# 3

# Growing Pains and Butterflies

*Puberty*

One sunny afternoon, Amy comes into my consulting room in the outpatient department at Amsterdam University Medical Center. She's thirty-two years old and relatively tall for a woman, at six-foot three. Amy has been sent by her husband, who noticed changes to her face. Over the past few years, her nose and ears have grown distinctly bigger and her chin more pronounced. Amy explains that her feet have grown too and that she has difficulty speaking, as if her tongue is too big. She is really concerned now that her periods have stopped and she has started bumping into things, as if her right eye isn't working properly. She is also experiencing problems at work; she is often so tired that a full day's work is virtually impossible.

As an endocrinologist, these symptoms ring alarm bells. Further examination and a brain scan confirm my suspicions – Amy has a tumour in her pituitary gland that is producing too much growth hormone. The tumour is so large that it is pressing against the other parts of the pituitary gland, which is involved in reproduction and energy metabolism. This explains her loss of bodily functions. This is a clear example of how harmful overproduction of hormones can be for your whole body.

Everything turns out all right for Amy; an operation on her pituitary gland returns her growth hormone to the desired level. Her periods return, and she recently gave birth to a healthy baby boy.

Amy's case doesn't seem like a logical start to a chapter about puberty, but her story is enlightening. The tumour set all sorts of processes in motion in her body that also take place in puberty, although in puberty these processes happen in a natural and healthy way. Under the influence of growth hormone, adolescents grow. And soaring reproductive hormones cause them to develop sexually and to act more impulsively.

'Adolescence is a new birth, for the higher and more completely human traits are now born,' the evolutionary psychologist Granville Stanley Hall (1844–1924) wrote.[1] Growth takes centre stage during this period, which is why we use the word 'adolescence' (from the Latin *adolescere*, meaning 'to grow up') to describe that age. However, when it comes to developing from child into self-sufficient adult, there's more to it than simply getting taller. During puberty, a child also becomes fertile and their behaviour changes. It is likely that reproductive hormones and pheromones subconsciously play a much bigger role in our reproduction than we previously thought. Let's first look at how this fertility comes about.

# The start of sexual development

On average, puberty starts between the ages of eight and four-teen, but this hasn't always been the case. The age of onset of puberty is dropping steadily.[2] In the 1980s, the paediatrician Marcia Herman-Giddens revealed the shocking research find-ings that the first signs of a developing reproductive system were being seen ever earlier in both girls and boys.[3,4] It is hard to imagine, but the average age that a girl started menstruating (as the onset of puberty) in 1860 was 16.6 years. Studies from the seventeenth and eighteenth centuries show that it was com-pletely normal for menstruation to start only around the age of twenty.[5] Herman-Giddens was not the first to observe a shift in the reproductive age, and put it down to our changing diet, expo-sure to environmental pollution, chemicals and a high level of social stress. Which factors really influence the onset of puberty? People have been racking their brains about this for centuries.

When writing about animal reproduction in one of his major texts, *De partibus animalium* ('The Parts of Animals'), the Greek philosopher Aristotle (fourth century BC) suggested that we have the power to influence the timing of fertility in humans.[6] Contrary to today's view, a delayed onset of puberty was long considered a problem. To speed up the onset of puberty, women were encouraged to talk, kiss or engage in sexual activity with male peers. Almost four centuries ago, the British scientist Francis Bacon claimed that accelerated puberty was due to 'innate heat': early maturity as a result of warm environmental temperatures. As proof of this, he referred to the fact that girls in Spain and Turkey started their periods at a younger age than those in the Netherlands or Sweden. His claim was supported by the seventeenth-century doctor Georg Friedrich Rall, who had noticed that prostitutes started menstruating at a younger age.

He claimed that this was because they had a 'warmer temperament' with men around.[7]

The idea that a higher body temperature accelerates puberty remains a theory. One thing we do know is that over the past few centuries, our body temperature has decreased by about half a degree on average.[8] Hard physical work also contributes to a later onset of puberty. Women in the seventeenth, eighteenth and nineteenth centuries who carried out hard physical labour and had a lower body weight often started their periods considerably later than their well-nourished peers from higher social circles.[9]

In the eighteenth century, the French philosopher and writer Jean-Jacques Rousseau claimed that direct contact with the other sex wasn't necessary; romantic literature or music could also hasten the onset of menstruation. Livestock farmers must have agreed with him. With sheep and pigs, a male of the same species is often brought in to a group of female animals to stimulate their fertility. Physical contact is superfluous, since the pheromones do their job via the air, as mentioned earlier.[10]

Pheromones were also the subject of research carried out by psychologist Martha McClintock in 1971. She stumbled upon the phenomenon of 'menstrual synchrony', whereby the menstrual cycles of women who live together in close proximity start to synchronise under the influence of pheromones.[11] Despite a barrage of criticism about the interpretation of the results, her research put pheromones in the spotlight of the press. Further research revealed that odourless moisture from the armpits of women in the fertile phase of their cycle influenced the hormone levels of other women who were exposed to it.[12,13] The synchronisation of menses in women who live in the same household has admittedly not been fully proven in scientific terms, but it may well be recognisable to female readers.

## Bach and ever-earlier puberty in boys

Lots has been written about the age at which girls get their first period and their hormonal maturation begins. But what about boys? This knowledge remained hidden for years until, in the 1960s, the medical historian S. F. Daw from the University of Oxford thought to look in an unexpected place: among students of Johann Sebastian Bach.[14] The famous German Baroque composer worked at St Thomas School in Leipzig between 1723 and 1750, where he led a number of boys' choirs. This boarding school took the musical activities of its pupils very seriously and meticulously noted down which pupils sung the high and low parts. Daw discovered that this depended on whether or not the pupils' voices had broken. Sopranos' voices had not yet broken, altos were in a period of transition and tenors' and basses' voices had already broken.

While voice-break cannot be taken as the start of puberty, it does give an indication of the average age this period begins: sixteen-and-a-half to seventeen years. When Daw published his study in 1970, English boys' voices broke at the average age of 13.3 years, down from 18 years at the start of the eighteenth century, and their puberty started even earlier. This suggests that the onset of puberty in boys, like girls, is constantly falling.

It is clear that many factors influence our complex endocrine system. This makes it difficult to establish the exact role they play in the early onset of puberty.

## Raging hormones and doing stupid things

During puberty, your body changes, but so too does your behaviour. The Dutch professor Jelle Jolles offers parents a helping hand when it comes to dealing with teenage children in his book *Het tienerbrein* ('The Teenage Brain').[15] In it, he advocates creating conditions for personal growth, so teenagers can gain new experiences within set boundaries. His advice is: be a coach who provides feedback and inspiration, as opposed to a referee. And keep talking to your children, even if it sometimes feels like a one-way conversation.

It's unsurprising that people associate adolescence with a certain kind of behaviour; the teenage years go hand in hand with a bomb of sex hormones, whereby testosterone and oestrogen start surging through the adolescent body. Spots, body odour (sweat!), sudden beard growth, emotional instability and not knowing what to do with your limbs that have grown out of proportion (let alone the first wet dream) – does this all sound familiar? Those raging hormones don't generally make adolescence an easy period, but like all natural processes, these ups and downs have an important function for the development of your brain and the rest of your body.

Puberty is the period in which you sexually 'mature'. Oestrogen stimulates breast development and menstruation in girls, whereas testosterone triggers beard growth, the production of sperm cells and muscle mass in boys. Mother Nature still sees having and raising children as one of the main tasks of our time here on earth, so it's essential to be both physically and mentally prepared for the responsibility. As not all parts of the brain develop at the same rate, you lose your balance during puberty; the activities of your emotional 'reward centre' (limbic system) and your rational 'planning centres' (prefrontal cortex) are not aligned. Put simply, your mind is less active than your emotions. The bigger the difference between the two, the more impulsive and the riskier the adolescent's behaviour.

Impulsivity is an interesting issue for researchers all over the world. In the documentary *Braintime* (2016), the developmental psychologist Eveline Crone asks how it makes sense for a brain that is developing to simultaneously do 'stupid things'.[16] While it's not only adolescents who favour short-term pleasure and make illogical decisions, adolescence is the period in which addiction problems can arise.

Hormones seem to hold sway here too. More testosterone in the blood (in boys and girls) stimulates the already-active reward centre. In the brain testosterone impairs the connection between the gland involved in recognising danger and the region that helps make decisions.[17] An American study showed, for example, that adolescent girls (between the ages of ten and fourteen) took more financial risks as the testosterone levels in their blood increased.[18] In a different study, adult men were administered testosterone. These men were more likely than members of the control group to make incorrect intuitive decisions as opposed to well-considered ones.[19]

Risk-taking, experimentation with alcohol and drugs, and other 'socially undesirable' behaviours in adolescents can be partially explained by those rising testosterone levels. Testosterone has a huge impact; research shows that even exposure to testosterone during pregnancy can have far-reaching consequences. The higher your testosterone levels as a foetus, the more risks, including financial ones, you are likely to take when older.[20]

It's important to view adolescent behaviour as a natural process and not to respond to it with punishment or criticism. That said, we know it's not just biological factors and upbringing that influences the behaviour of teenagers but also the culture in which a child grows up.[21] When the American anthropologist Margaret Mead studied the behaviour of young people in Samoa, a Polynesian island, in the 1920s, she concluded that teenagers behaved differently in that culture and that the above-mentioned stereotypical behaviour was not universal; that it perhaps depended more on 'nurture' than 'nature', though it's worth adding that Mead's methodology was highly controversial.

Perhaps it puts things into perspective to know that impulsive behaviour is not just a product of our times; increasing levels of 'problem behaviour' appears common to all eras. At the start of the sixteenth century, the French poet Bourbon wrote, 'A thirteen-year-old boy today is more deceptive and engages in more questionable practices than ten burly boys from our parents' day and age. The same can be said of girls. What could be the cause of this? Children today are maturing earlier.'[22]

We must also ask ourselves whether the impulsive behaviour is really so undesirable in adolescents. This may be the case in the short term, but in the long term, unruly adolescents tend to be more helpful and get more pleasure out of cooperating with others when they are older. Perhaps socially desirable behaviour can develop more in a brain left to grow and explore boundaries. Try looking at a difficult, contrary child that way. They might just be practising their emotional intelligence.[23]

---

### The marshmallow experiment: about impulsivity in children and adolescents

In the mid-1950s, the clinical psychologist Walter Mischel made a chance discovery. He was staying in a region with

---

people of East-Indian and African-American descent, who accused each other of greed and impulsivity respectively. Mischel wondered whether these groups did, in fact, differ in their ability to delay gratification. He carried out an initial version of the now-famous marshmallow experiment.

Children of various ages were offered a marshmallow. He gave them two choices: you can either eat the marshmallow immediately, or wait a couple of minutes and you will get two. Not all children (of the same age) were equally capable of delaying gratification. The clips that can be found online show some children stuffing the marshmallow into their mouths immediately, while others sit on their own hands so they can't touch it.[24]

Upon returning to the US, Mischel standardised his marshmallow test into a fully-fledged experiment, which he carried out at his daughters' primary school in collaboration with Stanford University. Years later, he determined that the children who were able to delay gratification (and resist the marshmallow) were slightly more successful at school and in their careers when they were older. Although recent repeat experiments have shown that these conclusions might not be as clear-cut as initially thought, this test still captures the imagination today.[25] This has led, for example, to a socially responsible episode of *Sesame Street*, in which the Cookie Monster teaches self-control (see YouTube: 'Me want it, but me wait'). You can even buy T-shirts with the slogan DON'T EAT THE MARSHMALLOW on them!

# Butterflies and heartbreak: sexual attraction

You may have noticed that adolescents can consume huge quantities of food without gaining weight. This is remarkable, especially because they tend to love junk food and sugary drinks.[26] Even after having wolfed down their dinners, my teenage kids complain that they are still hungry and grab a packet of crisps.

Besides an insatiable appetite, other processes also take place in their stomachs: namely butterflies when falling in love and nausea when experiencing heartbreak. The cuddle hormone prolactin and the mood hormone serotonin play a key role here. Ninety-five per cent of the body's serotonin is produced in the gut and can influence the movement of the intestines as well as gut feeling.[27]

Sexual attraction mainly takes place via your body – your brain doesn't have much say in the matter. The assumption that the man is often the seducer is questionable. A woman can also use her body language to show that she wants to be seduced. That's how the married couple Allan and Barbara Pease explain all sorts of non-verbal cues that women transmit in their book *Why Men Don't Listen and Women Can't Read Maps*.[28]

Our pheromones and hormones play an important role in this 'dance of love'. During flirtation and seduction, the dopamine level in your blood rises.[29] This focuses your attention, increases your heart rate, improves your mood and makes you feel good about yourself. The stress hormone cortisol also plays a role in seduction, and it has a different effect in men and women. If you are a woman with a high level of stress hormone in your blood, you are less receptive to attempts of seduction, whereas stressed men are more open to it; perhaps through the prospect of lovemaking as a quick way to relieve stress.[30]

And then there's the first kiss, which is also crucial for what happens next. Besides dopamine, kissing also releases oxytocin, which provides a pleasant feeling. But that doesn't mean that everything is all right. A recent, large-scale study showed that 50 per cent of women who were first attracted to a partner on the basis of appearance lost interest after a few kisses.[31] While only 15 per cent of women indicated that they would want to have sex with a man they hadn't kissed, most men reported that they wouldn't have a problem with a sexual partner whose saliva they hadn't yet tasted. This difference can be explained by the different types and concentrations of hormones in the saliva of men and women. Under the influence of oestrogens (involved in the menstrual cycle), women can send messages about their fertility via their saliva. Around the time of ovulation, for example, saliva contains more sugar, so a woman's kisses literally taste sweeter at this time.[32] Men who smell vulvar and axillary (underarm) odours collected from women around the time of ovulation have higher levels of testosterone in their saliva within one hour,[33] which increases their sexual desire. In both cases, the exchange of saliva through kissing can encourage the subconscious mind to reproduce.

Women therefore appear to use kissing primarily as a way to help them find a suitable partner. This evolutionary trick works as follows: a woman instinctively chooses a man who forms the best genetic match with her so that they can create as many healthy offspring as possible.[34] This is a partner who has different genetic features as this will make the offspring stronger. In order for the profiles to be a good match in genetic terms, nature enlists the help of pheromones.

This is an example of wonderful teamwork between the belly, hormones and brain, even if the contraceptive pill appears to impede the 'right' pheromone-driven choice of partner in women. Unfortunately we don't yet know exactly how this interference works.[35] And what are we to make of the effects of all the advertisements for fragrances that make you irresistible, passionfruit shower gels, and deodorants that stop you sweating for forty-eight hours? These developments make picking up on the cloud of pheromones a mission impossible. No longer being able to smell the person beside you on the rush-hour train is all well and good, but weigh this up against the consequences of a poor choice of partner. 'Fewer divorces thanks to limited deodorant use' would make a great headline, but of course it's all much more subtle than that.[36] After all, character traits are much more important motives for choosing a life partner than biology.

## The importance of growth hormone

An important characteristic of puberty is the growth spurt. The responsible hormone (human growth hormone or HGH) is one of the most recently discovered hormones; its existence was only uncovered in 1955, in Professor Choh Hao Li's lab at the University of California.[37] Li discovered eight of the nine major hormones produced by the pituitary gland, including follicle-stimulating hormone (FSH) and luteinising hormone (LH), both mentioned earlier. Growth hormone is less important in adulthood, but it plays a crucial role in puberty. This hormone, produced by the pituitary gland, ensures that a newborn baby measuring twenty inches grows to the size of an adult. With an ultimate height of between five and six-and-a-half feet, our height triples or quadruples in the first eighteen years of our lives.

When you're young, growth hormone ensures you grow in height by sending out signals to the growth plates in the long bones of your skeleton. In adults, growth hormone plays a different role. It helps you burn a high-fat meal more easily so you don't gain too much weight.[38] It also converts glycogen into glucose, thereby raising your blood sugar level and releasing energy. Growth hormone also increases your muscle mass, supports heart function and wound healing, and even has a positive effect on your mood.

And, as we saw earlier, everything is interconnected where hormones are concerned. If too little growth hormone is produced, your growth can stagnate and your muscle mass can decrease. This, in turn, influences your metabolism (how your body gets energy from the food you eat) and increases the likelihood of developing illnesses such as type 2 diabetes. Organs may start functioning less effectively as a result. In adults, this can lead to weight gain, less muscle strength, fatigue, weaker bones and high cholesterol. Research has shown that good sleep, plenty of exercise and fasting can positively influence the release of growth hormone and that stress has the opposite effect.

To return to height: children grow throughout their youth, but the biggest acceleration in growth is seen in the teenage years. In this period, more growth hormone is found in the blood. The pituitary gland sends growth hormone to the bloodstream in surges, about six times a day, with the highest levels observed at night. This is responsible for the growth spurt and the associated growing pains. In the Netherlands, women grow to an average of five-foot seven and men to six feet, making the Dutch among the tallest people in the world. This hasn't always been the case; until a hundred and fifty years ago, they were among the shortest Europeans.[39] What caused this change? It can perhaps be explained by the increased consumption of dairy products, as promoted by the government (children in western countries have been given milk at school since the 1950s). Frequent consumption of cows' milk has, in fact, been shown to increase levels of growth hormone in children.[40] Height also has a genetic advantage; taller, and therefore more muscular men are more attractive as partners from an evolutionary point of view and are also more fertile than their shorter peers.

In the event of normal growth, HGH is therefore released in surges. A continuously elevated level of this hormone is unusual. This is only seen if there is a tumour in the pituitary gland, as was the case with Amy. If this happens at a young age, the bones have not yet grown fully and the result is gigantism (more about this later). If excess growth hormones are emitted after puberty, we refer to this as acromegaly (enlarged limbs). This often leads to abnormally large hands, feet, jaw, nose and ears – features utilised by the Dutch actor Carel Struycken (seven feet tall and shoe size 18.5) for his role as Lurch in *The Addams Family*. This excessive growth disorder is present in around six in every hundred thousand people. While it's a rare condition, it's not uncommon among certain groups, such as basketball players, who are often selected for their height.[41] But it's not always possible to determine whether or not someone suffers from acromegaly based on their height alone; a hormone test is needed for this.

Gigantism is an extreme growth disorder that has been documented since ancient times. In the *Periplus*, the Ancient Greek version of Google Maps from around 6 BC, used by seafarers to find their way safely along the Atlantic coast of Europe,[42] the author describes the mysterious island of Albion, where an army of powerful women lived who reproduced with evil spirits and gave birth to giant children ('the sons of Anak'). The giants inhabited the island for hundreds of years, until Brutus of Troy arrived. Together with his soldiers, he conquered his 'Britainnia' by throwing the leader of the group of giants, Gogmagog, off a cliff. Brutus then founded New Troy. Albion is now known as Great Britain, which owes its name in part to Brutus, and New Troy is known as London.

Britain isn't unique when it comes to imaginative stories

about giants. Think, for example, of Goliath, the giant from the Bible who fought David, and of the children of Anak ('long neck') in Canaan. Hereditary gigantism was also seen in Roman imperium families.[43,44] The fact that there were really tall people all over the world has been proved by archaeological discoveries of human skeletons. Interestingly, all of these skeletons have a strikingly large *sella turcica* in the skull, the protective depression in which the pituitary gland is located. Perhaps these giants, like Amy, had enlarged pituitary glands, as a result of a tumour, that produced too much growth hormone.

The connection between gigantism and a malfunctioning pituitary gland was established after analysing the skeleton of the Irishman Charles Byrne, who was seven foot seven inches tall.[45] Byrne lived in London between 1761 and 1783 and performed at fairs as a type of 'Big Friendly Giant'. Like most giants, he died young, at the age of twenty-two; after his death, his skeleton was exhibited to the public in a museum. A good century later, this enabled the neurosurgeon and endocrinologist Harvey Cushing to diagnose his condition: according to Cushing, the gigantism caused by a tumour in the pituitary gland.

What's striking is that all of Charles Byrne's descendants were also extremely tall. We had to wait until 2009 for genetic proof that this type of gigantism was hereditary. Márta Korbonits, a professor of endocrinology in London, noticed that gigantism was more prevalent in Irish people who lived near Charles Byrne's place of birth. Márta and her research team isolated Byrne's DNA from the teeth of the skeleton, which was more than two hundred years old – a highly complex, technical undertaking. They then compared this DNA with that of the descendants of Charles Byrne who were still alive and ... bingo! They found a deviation in the DNA that was responsible for the exceptional height of the entire family.

It is unclear whether this mutation also played a role in the case of the Dutch girl Trijntje Keever (1616–33), nicknamed 'The Big Girl'. With a height of eight-foot four at the age of seventeen, she is the tallest woman ever documented.[46] We do know that Rigardus Rijnhout, nicknamed the 'Giant of Rotterdam' (1922–59), had a tumour in his pituitary gland. Weighing seventeen-and-a-half pounds at birth, he grew to a height of seven-foot nine inches, wore shoe size 29 and ended up weighing thirty-six stone! A statue of him was erected in Rotterdam in 2011.[47] The American Robert Wadlow, a contemporary of Rijnhout, is the tallest man ever, according to the *Guinness Book of Records*, which records his height as eight-foot eleven.

## Sleeping, exercising, eating and fasting

In the hormonal traffic, nighttime is rush hour. During deep sleep, our muscles relax, our blood pressure decreases and our breathing slows down. It is a phase of growth and recovery; new cells are produced and energy levels are replenished. It is predominantly during the deep, slow-wave sleep that growth hormones are delivered to the blood. It's just a shame that your typical adolescent isn't a fan of getting an early night. That said, considering most young people disregard virtually every unwritten rule about sleep, they often function surprisingly well.

### The Grand Grenadiers of Potsdam

In the mid-seventeenth century, the Prussian King Frederick William I was fascinated with exceptionally tall men – possibly because he was on the smaller side himself, measuring a stocky five-foot two inches. In 1668, he therefore put together a regiment of the Prussian army made up of recruits who were at least six-foot two inches. The Grand Grenadiers of Potsdam (also known as the Potsdam Giants) grew into a group of 3200 soldiers from the Ottoman and Russian army.[48] Friedrich attempted to marry off the men to tall women to create a race of giants. In 1740, after the king died, his son Frederick the Great disbanded the regiment. He was not convinced about an army of 'Long Guys', especially when it emerged they had never fought in a war.

This may be due to the fact that those slow waves predominantly occur in the first three hours of sleep in young people. A good quality of sleep in this short period is therefore, in principle, sufficient for recovery and for building muscle tissue. But you have to sleep in accordance with your biological clock, whose timings shift a fair bit during puberty. An adolescent who doesn't go to bed until late at night can sleep as long as they like, but because the quality of sleep they are getting is poor, their production of growth hormone is impacted.

The use of tablets and smartphones during evenings also throws a spanner in the works.[49] This creates a different sleep pattern and inhibits the production of melatonin (sleep hormone) from the pineal gland, which in turn inhibits the production of growth hormone.[50] Could this be one of the reasons why, for the first time, we are seeing a generation of Dutch people smaller than their parents?[51]

Physical activity also naturally stimulates the production and release of growth hormone. Movement stimulates muscle and cell growth, which in turn ensures that the adolescent's bones are strong. For young adults, running or jumping is more effective than walking or swimming.[52]

In the 1980s, athletes discovered that growth hormone supplements could improve performance and decrease the risk of long-term injury. Although the evidence was weak – unless the hormone was used in combination with testosterone – synthetic growth hormone became extremely popular with athletes and bodybuilders. In 1989, the International Olympic Committee listed human growth hormone as a banned substance, but because of a lack of effective screening opportunities (growth hormone cannot be detected in urine and can only be detected in blood between twenty-four and forty-eight hours after an injection), its use did not decrease. In fact, the 1996 Summer Olympics in Atlanta were nicknamed the 'Growth Hormone Games' due to the abundant use of human growth hormone during the event.[53]

Besides sleep and exercise, fasting is also a powerful stimulus for the increased production of growth hormone.[54] This may seem contradictory – why would a body grow without sufficient fuel? If your stomach is empty, ghrelin – also known as the 'hunger hormone' – is produced. The higher the level of ghrelin, the greater your appetite and sense of hunger. The name 'ghrelin' comes from growth-hormone-releasing peptides. What ghrelin does (among other things) during short-term hunger is boost the production of growth hormone,[55] increasing your blood sugar level and releasing energy to repair your body.

A popular type of fasting is intermittent fasting.[56] This is where you restrict the number of hours in which you eat during a day. You might, for example, fast from eight in the evening until noon the next day. More and more people are attempting long-term fasting based on various alleged health benefits (although these have not yet been scientifically proven).

Although moderate fasting has a positive effect on the production of growth hormone, the negative effects of extreme fasting can be seen in patients with anorexia. People with anorexia, who are often young, eat very little out of fear of gaining weight. As a result, they end up with chronic deficiencies and serious disturbances to their metabolism, including that of their bones and blood sugar levels,[57] comparable with the effects that the Dutch 'hunger winter' of 1944–45 had on the human body.

## Stress

While acute physical 'stress', as caused by intensive exercise, produces more growth hormone, long-term psychological stress can lead to a shortage of it. Children who experience chronic stress can fall behind in terms of their growth.[58] This rare condition is referred to as 'psychosocial dwarfism' – delayed growth without a physical cause – and occurs in children up to around the age of fifteen who grow up in a stressful environment, such as around domestic violence. This form of dwarfism is relatively unknown in the medical world, but is a feature of various fictional stories and films. In Victor Hugo's *Les Misérables*, for example, the eight-year-old Cosette is as small as a four-year-old due to her dreadful childhood, but she starts growing again once Jean Valjean adopts her.

Even if you try to 'turn on' the production of growth hormone in these children by synthetic means, the pituitary gland doesn't respond well. What does help is moving the child to a different, less stressful environment. If that happens, the hormone levels can recover, sometimes within just three weeks.[59]

If the cause of the growth hormone deficiency is physical, the shortage can be offset with synthetic growth hormone, but that has to be carried out carefully.

Around 1960, the aforementioned Professor Li, who discovered growth hormone, managed to filter growth hormone from the pituitary gland of human corpses. This somewhat gruesome method was used to obtain exogenous growth hormone until as recently as 1985. At that time, injecting children with growth hormone was seen as harmless and was carried out on a relatively large scale but, as is often the case in medical history, it was not without its consequences. The injections resulted in an increased risk of bowel cancer and the fatal Creutzfeldt-Jakob disease, as the disease was transferred to healthy recipients via the pituitary glands of donors who had succumbed to it.[60] Since then, doctors have switched to safe, biosynthetic variants developed by pharmaceutical companies, which are identical to the growth hormone that children produce themselves.

Growth hormone is an important hormone for children, and for burgeoning adolescents in particular. A shortage of it is apparent when growth is delayed, whereas too much of it can lead to gigantism. But the more subtle disorders related to growth hormone levels are harder to spot. What you can do as a parent is try to establish a number of simple rules for your teenager to follow: sufficient, good-quality sleep, daily exercise (half an hour a day), a varied diet, limited screen time before bed, and the avoidance of chronic stress (relaxation). As a father of three adolescents, I can only wish you the best of luck!

In the next chapter I will look more closely at how the interplay between hormones and brain development can determine our personality and even our preferred gender.

# 4

# Homosexuality and Transgender People

*About the Influence of Hormones on Our*
*Gender Identity and Sexual Preference*

Herman is a 45-year-old man from the tip of the Dutch province of North Holland. At a height of six-foot five and with a muscular physique – he has been a farmer virtually his entire life – he cuts an imposing figure. Manlier than manly, you might say: his handshake stings for a while in the palm of my hand after he enters my consulting room. In the safety of that space he explains that he has felt like a woman his entire life. He dislikes rough sports and has never played football. At home on the farm he wears women's clothes; that's the only time he ever feels at ease.

After his children flew the nest he decided to be true to himself and undergo gender reassignment surgery. He has the full support of his wife, who has also come with him to Amsterdam.

I first met Herman in 2010 during my endocrinology placement at the VU University Medical Center, now part of

Amsterdam University Medical Center, which has become a leading authority in the field of transgender healthcare. Many stories like Herman's can be found in Alex Bakker's *Transgender in the Netherlands*, which is well worth a read.[1] A common feature in these stories, covering the past seventy years, is a feeling of being born in the wrong body, also known as 'gender dysphoria', and the ensuing psychological distress.

As human beings were traditionally divided into two sexes – male and female – binary thinking was dominant for a long time. A man was defined by having XY chromosomes, a penis and testes, a certain body composition and lots of testosterone, whereas women had the following characteristics: XX chromosomes, a vagina, ovaries, a womb and the presence of lots of oestrogen. This distinction was based on sex hormones. Sex refers to the biological difference between people, i.e. the physical characteristics with which someone is born, whereas gender includes the cultural and psychological aspects of what it means to be a man or woman.[2] A common explanation is: sex is what's between your legs and gender is what's between your ears. Intersex is the biological term for a body with both male and female sexual characteristics, like that of the runner Foekje Dillema or the Dutch rock star Raven van Dorst.

This binary thinking led to the assumption that transgender people (people whose gender identity or experience doesn't correspond with their biological sex) and homosexual people (people who are attracted to people of the same sex) display unnatural behaviour. But a look at nature sheds a different light on the matter.

In the animal kingdom, around 5 to 6 per cent of populations display an interest in a partner of the same sex. Homosexuality has been widely documented in more than 65,000 animal species, including birds, insects, primates, dolphins and the penguins at Amsterdam's Artis Zoo, all of whom display regular sexual behaviour with members of the same sex.[4] But the difference between homosexuality in humans and animals is that animals that exhibit homosexual behaviour often reproduce with a member of the opposite sex.[5] In the plant world, hermaphroditism is the norm.[6] Certain animal species, like the clownfish featured in the Disney film *Finding Nemo*, can switch sex during their lifetime. Sea bass can even assume both sexes. According to biologists, they do this to prevent the group from consisting of too many males or females: an imbalance which would threaten their survival.[7] There are plenty of examples in nature of animals adapting their behaviour under the influence of various sex hormones.

Gender fluidity among humans is known all over the world and has always existed, the London-based historian Alicia Spencer-Hall claims in *Trans and Genderqueer Subjects in Medieval Hagiography* (2021).[8] According to Spencer-Hall, there are examples of men becoming women and vice versa all over the world. In contrast to the gender binary, the Bugis people from the Indonesian island of Sulawesi recognise five genders: cisgender men and cisgender women (whose gender identity corresponds with their sex at birth), transgender men and transgender women, and intersex people, reserved for spiritual leaders like priests or shamans. Spencer-Hall also describes a monk, Brother Joseph, who lived as a transgender man almost eight centuries ago and was declared a saint by the Church. How differently things turned out for Pope Joan (see Chapter 1).

In this chapter I will first discuss the biological background of gender identity before looking at how our sexual orientation is formed. I will end by discussing our relationship with our sex hormones.

## When he's a she and she's a he

It's estimated that 0.3 to 0.6 per cent of the western population is transgender, with more transgender women (women who were born as men) than transgender men.[9] In total, there are around fifty thousand transgender people in the Netherlands who have accessed medical health care, but it's not known how many have had gender reassignment surgery.

Since the 1980s, the level of acceptance towards transgender people in most countries has increased, especially in Western Europe. Unfortunately, however, there are still some countries, such as those in Eastern Europe and Africa, that have only become less tolerant in this regard.[10] Even in the Netherlands, the forced coming-out of YouTuber and make-up artist Nikkie de Jager in 2020 showed that taboos around gender identity and biological sex still exist.[11] Although many people were surprised that this story made the news, the seventeen-minute monologue by Nikkie Tutorials – as the influencer refers to herself – has been viewed millions of times on her YouTube channel. She didn't make her statement voluntarily, but as a result of being blackmailed. Thanks to role models like her, it is becoming more accepted that preadolescent children express their gender identity, and increasing numbers of them are doing just that.

Research shows that 57 per cent of the Dutch population has a positive perception of transgender people.[12] Dutch TV programmes like *Geslacht!* ('Sex!'), *Hij is een Zij* ('He is a She') and *Love Me Gender* have contributed to this, as have older examples like Dana International, who won the Eurovision Song Contest for Israel in 1998, Kelly van der Veer from *Big Brother* and, more recently, Caitlyn Jenner, known from the reality series *The*

*Kardashians*, and Loiza Lamers, the winner of *Holland's Next Top Model*, who both came out in 2015.

---

### Pink for boys, blue for girls

Although it is a rather outdated concept, blue is still seen as a colour for boys and pink for girls. However, this was the other way round for a long time – until relatively recently, in fact.

In 1918, a well-known American magazine published a 'guideline': pink was the colour for boys, and blue for girls.[13] It was the first time that colours had been associated with a sex, possibly inspired by the many religious depictions of baby Jesus dressed in red/pink and Mary in blue. After the Second World War, this trend abruptly reversed. There are various theories as to why this happened, but it is possible that it was a response to the uniforms worn by women during the war. In the 1950s, the American First Lady Mamie Eisenhower set the tone by wearing a tremendous pink inaugural gown.[14] Many others followed her lead, including the 'pink ladies' in *Grease* and the 'plastics' in *Mean Girls*, and Hillary Clinton frequently chooses the colour pink when attending meetings about strengthening the position of women.

British research has shown that adults have a preference for blues, but that women respond more positively to mixtures with red hues and men to those with green.[15] In the 1920s and 1930s, 'Das lila Lied' ('The Lavender Song') was the signature song of the German gay and lesbian movement.[16] In the last century, Oscar Wilde wore a green carnation to acknowledge his sexual preference, whereas a red tie was seen as a sign of homosexuality in the US.

---

Dutch children are now calling for less strict divisions. Twelve-year-old Julia, for example, contacted the Dutch department store HEMA via Facebook to ask if they would stock less girly girls' clothes.[17] HEMA thought it was a good idea and decided to merge the 'boys' and 'girls' sections to form the gender-neutral 'kids' section.

To the outside world, someone is only transgender after their transition, whereas for the transgender person themselves the identity is not new; the transition just marks the end of their development. *Valentijn*, the wonderful documentary by Hetty Nietsch, shows how Valentijn transitions from boy to girl in a society that is predominantly binary and in which you are seen as either 'man' or 'woman'. These strict attitudes explain one of the reasons why depression is almost three times as prevalent in young transgender people than in the general population. Transgender people are also bullied more often than their peers and are more likely to be emotionally neglected or abused at home.[18] A fear of confrontation and possible blackmail often hangs over them like a sword of Damocles.

Doctors are getting better at knowing when and how best to carry out hormonal and surgical interventions, and how best to provide psychological support. As there are considerable waiting lists in the Netherlands and the process itself can take between one and two years, there is no longer one set path offered for everyone. Some people may only want hormones, while others want gender reassignment surgery, which is irreversible. At the start of the century, doctors started prescribing puberty blockers to patients after stringent psychological screening. Puberty blockers inhibit the physical changes of puberty in girls and boys, and they marked a significant milestone for the acceptance and emancipation of transgender people. Nikkie de Jager, for example, received hormone treatment from the age of fourteen and had surgery before twenty. As teenagers who receive these hormone treatments do not develop any secondary sexual characteristics (such as breasts or beard growth), they are spared the associated suffering both physically and psychologically. Early treatment leads to better results from a cosmetic point of view than treatment as an adult, as with my patient Herman. Her wife and children fully accepted Herman's transition. She is still in good physical health and is delighted with the final result.

Greater life satisfaction is an important success factor; after transitioning, both adults as well as teenagers value their lives just as much as their cisgender peers; the percentage of transgender people who regret the surgery is negligible.[19] Acceptance and support from parents during the transition process also increase self-esteem.[20]

## Early examples of transgender people

There are many examples of famous transgender people throughout history, such as Elagabalus, a Roman emperor from the second century AD, who frequently wore women's clothing and supposedly offered a vast sum of money to any doctor who could provide him with a vagina.[21] Some well-known historical figures, such as Joan of Arc (1412–31) and Queen Christina of Sweden (1626–89),[22] are also considered to have been transgender. It wasn't until 1912 that the surgeon Richard Mühsam removed the breasts and ovaries of an anonymous transgender man in Berlin. Eight years later, Mühsam performed gender reassignment surgery, again on an anonymous person.[23] This intervention is officially considered the first gender reassignment operation.

In the 1950s, a former soldier hit the headlines as a transgender woman. George Jorgensen was born in New York during the Roaring Twenties. He was a shy boy who didn't fit in at school and was often bullied and called gay. After completing military service, he signed up to study at the Medical and Dental Assistant School in Manhattan. In 1951, he started taking oestrogen supplements. He initially planned to have surgery in Sweden – the only country in the world to perform gender reassignment surgery at that time. However, George's relatives told him about Dr Christian Hamburger from Statens Serum Institute in Copenhagen, who experimented with sex hormone therapy. This doctor was happy to help George with both hormonal and surgical treatments,[24] as long as George allowed him to write a scientific report about it, as he did with 464 patients that followed.[25]

And so it came to pass: in October 1951, both of George's testicles were removed and one year later the penis was also removed. Unfortunately the Danish team of surgeons didn't yet have the technical expertise to construct a new vagina, but that was done later in the United States. And that is how Christine Jorgensen ended up on the front page of the *New York Daily News* in 1952 with the headline 'EX GI BECOMES BLONDE BEAUTY' and the world became acquainted with transgender people. Dr Hamburger subsequently received requests from hundreds of people all over the world for this type of treatment.

Christine became a celebrity; she starred in films and performed as a singer in nightclubs, but also became a role model. As a speaker on the subject of transsexuality, she called tirelessly for a greater acceptance, right up to her death in 1989. Transgender women in the US were, for a long time, referred to as 'Christines'.

# The transgender brain

In the 1970s, thanks to the medical advances helping people to change gender, a debate arose in the scientific world about the possible explanations for the phenomenon of gender dysphoria. Some doctors believed that a transgender identity was the result of strongly suppressed homoerotic feelings and should be treated as a psychiatric illness; psychoanalysis could be a way to achieve self-acceptance. Others believed that the cause was biological: perhaps the brain developed differently in transgender people.

One of the scientists who has long believed gender identity was linked to brain anatomy was the Dutch professor Dick Swaab. With the help of the Netherlands Brain Bank, he has spent many decades researching neurological changes via postmortem studies of people with certain sexual preferences and gender identities. In 1995, he demonstrated that a specific structure in the brain, the bed nucleus of the stria terminalis (BNST),[26] plays a critical role in gender identity. The BNST is larger in men than women, but Swaab discovered that transgender women, i.e. those who were born male, had smaller BNSTs than those of the average man in the study. In fact, they were about the same size as those born female.

One of Swaab's co-authors, Emeritus Professor Louis Gooren, contributed significantly to the professionalisation of transgender healthcare and the acceptance of transgender people in the Netherlands. He helped establish the transgender policy at Amsterdam's University Medical Center. Swaab's publication, as well as legislation – such as the Dutch Transgender Act of 1985, which allows transgender people to change their gender designation on their birth certificate – caused a snowball effect. Evidently, a biological basis was needed in order to achieve further acceptance. While the Dutch Transgender Act of 1985 was subject to a number of conditions, such as modifying the body to align with the desired gender and a sterilisation procedure, these requirements were abolished in 2014 with the amendment of the Transgender Act. This helped increase self-determination for transgender people.[27]

Although the majority of Dutch people view transgender people positively, a quarter have an issue with transsexuality and for 5 per cent of the Dutch population it would constitute a reason to terminate a friendship.[28] Social factors like these are slowing down the emancipation of transgender people; on average, transgender people have a lower income and are more likely to be lonely.[29] In the years prior to 2014, a change to the gender registration was made an average of eighty times a year; in 2015, 770 changes were made, and by 2017 this number had increased to 850.

Special gender clinics have existed in Amsterdam and Groningen since the 1970s and doctors there are struggling to keep up with demand. As the number of new patients is constantly increasing, additional gender clinics have since been set up in the Netherlands. Besides gender reassignment surgery, these specialist centres also offer psychological support and hormone therapies, which aim to enable a person's secondary sexual characteristics to better correspond with their gender identity.[30]

With his photo series *Inner Journey: Into Manhood*, the Dutch photographer Marvel Harris beautifully documented his transition from woman to man.[31] The Dutch philosopher and writer Maxim Februari also wanted to show through his book *The Making of a Man* that a transition can be a success story.[32] Maxim was born in 1963 as Marjolein Februari and started treatment for gender reassignment in the spring of 2012 after a long internal struggle. His personal notes about the use of testosterone and the associated physical effects are astonishing.[33] Physically, testosterone had a rejuvenating effect on Maxim's body, suddenly preventing the approaching menopause. His muscle strength increased, he grew out of his clothes and was constantly hungry. When his voice also deepened, his 'second puberty' was complete. Apart from having to get used to a different body, he also noticed emotional changes: he reacted more directly and got annoyed more quickly, but he could also shake off emotions more easily than before. Maxim, like many transgender men, also noticed that he started crying less and no longer lay awake worrying at night. Incidentally, the opposite also generally holds true: transgender women often report that they cry more once they start taking oestrogen.

Before his transition, Februari already referred to himself as a feminist; this conviction has only strengthened since then.[34] Despite increasing social understanding that gender is not a binary concept, he can confirm from his own experience that society treats men and women differently. Although it is a physically demanding process, the treatment of transgender people can therefore not only be seen as a liberation, but also as a fascinating phenomenon that enriches our medical knowledge and can be of great significance for patients with endocrine disorders.

As previously mentioned, transgender people are common to all times and cultures; the only thing that is strange is therefore society's negative response to them. Or, as Maxim Februari puts it: 'Gone are the times when we could make do with the contours of the body to describe the spirit within them.'[35]

# LGBTQI+

In (pre)adolescence, sexual and gender preferences develop alongside the reproductive organs. While games at primary school often have a 'girls vs. boys' element, it's usually not until secondary school that children start showing an interest in the opposite sex. A smaller number, however, become interested in members of their own sex. The term used to describe this is homosexuality (*homo* is Ancient Greek for 'same') and it is the opposite of heterosexuality (*hetero* is Ancient Greek for 'other'). The term homosexuality encompasses both gay and lesbian people. Incidentally, the term 'lesbian' goes back to Sappho, a Greek poet from the island of Lesbos who wrote numerous poems about erotic love between women. A more inclusive umbrella term is LGBTQI+, which refers to people who identify as lesbian, gay, bisexual, transgender, queer or intersex, with the + referring to all fluid, pan- or asexual people.

It's not yet clear how sexuality develops in people. We do know that a group of hormones called androgens leads to a masculinisation of the foetus. Exposure to these hormones (of which testosterone is the best-known) during pregnancy leads to the development of male sex organs, and later also to the 'masculinisation' of body and brain. Although there's no conclusive evidence that sex hormones influence the formation of an LGBTQI+ identity, there are indications that certain nuclei may play a role. Almost thirty years ago, Professor Dick Swaab and his research team discovered a part of the brain called the sexually dimorphic nucleus (SDN): a small group of neurons close to the hypothalamus responsible for controlling the production of sex hormones as well as our sexual behaviour.[36]

## Brain

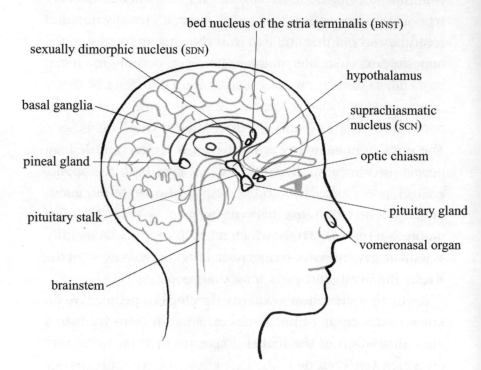

bed nucleus of the stria terminalis (BNST)

sexually dimorphic nucleus (SDN)

hypothalamus

basal ganglia

suprachiasmatic nucleus (SCN)

pineal gland

optic chiasm

pituitary stalk

pituitary gland

vomeronasal organ

brainstem

As mentioned earlier, this nucleus is bigger in men than in women. A few years later, Swaab turned his attention to another nucleus,[37] the suprachiasmatic nucleus (SCN), which may be involved in our sexual preferences and choice of sexual partners. The SCN appears to be influenced by pheromones, which are passed between people through the air and by touch, transmitting signals to our brain. In women and homosexual men – but not heterosexual men – the SCN responds to the male pheromone androstadienone.[38] Vice versa, in lesbian women this nucleus responds to female pheromones such as estratetraenol.[39]

In bisexual people, it appears to respond to both pheromones.[40]

Swaab's findings suggest that a gay or lesbian brain resembles that of the other sex, resulting in a preference for the same sex. It's unlikely, however, that there is such a clear dividing line.[41] Instead the development of sexual and gender preference is probably the result of the complex interplay between human body and the environment in which a person grows up.

## The influence of environmental factors

It may seem obvious to conclude that exposure to hormones during pregnancy can impact certain nuclei involved in sexual preference. A 1972 study exposed pregnant rats to chronic stress. These rats had high levels of the stress hormone cortisol in their bodies and their male offspring were more likely to exhibit male sexual behaviour than female.[42] Of course, the findings of these studies cannot simply be translated to humans. We can't (yet) estimate the effects of hormone fluctuations in the womb on human offspring. That said, exposure to chronic stress does appear to be associated with an increased risk of lifelong changes to health, even permanently altering certain genes.[43] Chronic stress makes the mother's adrenal gland produce continually elevated levels of the stress hormone cortisol, to which the foetus is exposed in the womb. As a result, the foetus's daily rhythm of hormone secretion goes haywire and the body becomes accustomed to the cortisol, which then causes the level of this hormone to increase.

The above-mentioned study on rats revealed that there are critical periods during pregnancy when elevated levels of stress hormone may have negative long-term effects on the foetus. It also showed that exposure to chronically high levels of cortisol in the blood caused testosterone levels in male offspring to decrease to levels more commonly seen in female rats.

There is still a huge stigma surrounding atypical sexual orientation. In many countries, this goes hand in hand with social exclusion. Those who oppose homosexuality often claim that it is unnatural, but it also occurs in the animal kingdom; homosexual relationships are commonly observed in bonobos, for example, as the biologist Frans de Waal established on various occasions.[44] The other species of animal in which this behaviour is exhibited to the same degree is the domestic sheep; on average, 8 to 10 per cent of rams prefer a relationship with another ram, irrespective of the number of ewes present.[45]

Almost ninety years ago, researchers noticed that boys with older brothers were more likely to be homosexual as adults.[46] Various studies followed confirming this observation: 15 to 30 per cent of all homosexual men had an older brother.[47] Strikingly, this only applied to biological brothers; sisters, half-brothers or adopted brothers made no difference.[48] Vice versa, a recent study carried out by Professor Henny Bos on the well-being of a large group of children with lesbian parents (whose development was followed for thirty years from birth) revealed that they weren't any more likely to be homosexual than children with heterosexual parents.[49]

Scientists are not entirely sure why homosexuality is more prevalent in families with older brothers. They suspect that the mother's immune system is involved.[50] If a mother is pregnant with a boy, the testosterone level in the womb is elevated and her immune system produces more antibodies against testosterone, so that future brothers release less of this hormone.[51] This could influence the formation of regions of the brain involved in sexual orientation. But this is only a theory; hard proof of the 'maternal immune hypothesis' has not yet been found.

In 1996, an updated hypothesis was put forward: for every

pregnancy with a boy, the mother is exposed to the H-Y anti-gen, which is specific to male cells.[52] As this is perceived by the mother as foreign matter, her immune system responds by pro-ducing antibodies. In every subsequent pregnancy with a boy, more and more of these antibodies reach the foetus through the placenta, where they influence the prenatal development of the brain. In order to test this theory, pregnant mice were vaccinated against the H-Y antigen in order to stimulate the production of antibodies.[53] A follow-up study on male baby mice revealed that they had very little sexual interest in female peers when they reached adulthood. However, the fact that the majority of homo-sexual men don't have a whole army of older brothers means that the maternal immune hypothesis at best describes one of the many environmental factors involved in the development of our sexual orientation.

# 5

# Old Choices in a New Paradise

*Obesity, Hunger and Hormones*

Thirty-five-year-old Maria comes into my consulting room one afternoon with her two young children in tow. She is having financial difficulties and her eyes well up when she tells me about it. She works night shifts in a care home in order to stay afloat. As a result, she is so tired by the time the weekend comes around that she doesn't have the energy to do anything, and she has barely any friends left. Her self-confidence has plummeted. She smokes to help alleviate the stress, and rarely exercises as she has constant pain in all her joints.

A miserable life for such a young woman. Her GP referred her to me after diagnosing her with type 2 diabetes, which is my specialist field. The question, of course, was how I could help her. We could use diabetes medication to slow down the effects, but we wouldn't be doing anything about the cause. Her main problem was that she weighed twenty stone.

Obesity is a growing problem in our western world. It prevents the cells in the pancreas that produce insulin from doing their job properly. The body then becomes less sensitive to insulin, which can ultimately lead to diabetes.

But what causes obesity in the first place? And how do people experience it?

This chapter will deal with hunger, obesity and hormones. To address these topics we first need to understand how we, as people, are programmed to deal with hunger and how our body protects us against food shortages. These primal mechanisms don't always match our modern lifestyles. Because of this, many people not only put on too much weight, but also keep that weight on. I will show how your gut is connected with your brain – an ingenious and fascinating construct, but one that can unfortunately also lead to complex eating behaviour.

## Obesity through the ages

Descriptions of obesity can be found throughout human history. The Old Testament tells the story of the obese King Eglon, who fell victim to an assassination. A sword entered his belly and disappeared in the enormous layer of fat. Obesity was particularly prevalent in royal households. The best-known example is the German Princess Caroline of Brandenburg-Ansbach, who became queen of England in the early eighteenth century.[1] She had become so fat that she could only turn over in bed with the help of her ladies-in-waiting. Although she was never depicted to the full extent in her portraits, her enormous breasts were world-famous. Beauty ideals change with the times; think of the large women that Rubens painted. Bearing this in mind, it's perhaps not surprising that Queen Caroline was so proud of her body that residents of London would buy tickets to watch her feasting in her palace on Sundays.

# The Power of Hormones

The clergy of the Middle Ages listed seven deadly sins including gluttony, sloth and wrath – a combination which appears in various religious texts. Pope Innocent VIII, for example, was known for his immense size.[2] He would spend the whole day sleeping and had a very unpleasant character. It was he who incited the witch hunts that led to innocent people being burned alive. He ultimately became so fat and so tired that he could no longer move around. Allegedly, he received blood transfusions from healthy boys as a form of treatment. Whether or not that's true, it was to no avail; both Pope Innocent VIII and the blood donors died.

With today's medical knowledge, we can see that the combination of obesity and fatigue experienced by Pope Innocent VIII corresponds with the symptoms of obstructive sleep apnoea syndrome (OSAS): a sleep disorder caused by obesity, whereby breathing stops for more than thirty seconds, several times a night. People with this disorder are unable to get deep enough REM sleep, which makes them feel drowsy, fatigued and grumpy during the day. The English prime minister Winston Churchill, who was well known for his mood swings and his size, also suffered from this. OSAS can also exacerbate diabetes. It also leads to an increased appetite, creating a vicious circle of obesity and sleep deprivation.

This has been the subject of research by the Belgian Professor Eve van Cauter for several decades now. She demonstrated that obesity and type 2 diabetes result in poor, short nighttime sleep.[3] In an experiment, she showed that short sleepers have lower concentrations of the satiety hormone leptin, which signals to the brain that you have eaten enough, and higher concentrations of the hunger hormone ghrelin. In addition, short sleepers are more likely to be attracted to meals that are high in fats and sugars. It's hardly surprising then that short sleep can, in the long term, lead to obesity and ultimately OSAS.

Incidentally, the best-known patient with this condition was described by Charles Dickens in *The Pickwick Papers* (1837).[4] The character Joe had these exact characteristics and that's why OSAS is sometimes referred to as 'Pickwickian syndrome'.

## An increasingly weighty problem

However sad their story may be, overweight people can generally expect limited understanding from their slimmer counterparts, who often wonder how someone can let things get that far. In their eyes, overweight people aren't patients with 'real' illnesses like cancer, gallstones or a broken hip – conditions that anyone can suffer from. But obesity, too, is a real condition.

In her book *Knap voor een dik meisje* ('Pretty for a Fat Girl'), published in 2019, Tatjana Almuli describes her battle with weight.[5] In 2015, she took part in the reality TV show *Obese* and lost around nine stone in ten months, but she continued receiving negative comments about her appearance and size. Scientific studies (and popular weight-loss programmes on TV) reveal that only 30 per cent of obese people who make a serious attempt to lose weight under strict supervision manage to continue eating less in the long term. Tatjana didn't belong to that group. The message in her book is clear: don't judge overweight people too harshly in a part of the world and at a time in which slim is the norm.

Despite that norm, almost every other adult in the Netherlands is overweight. Half of these are obese, posing a threat to their health. In total, one in six adults in the Netherlands end up with type 2 diabetes.

Let's return to Maria. Due to her weight, she is at increased risk of developing type 2 diabetes at a young age. But that's not all:

she is also more susceptible to high cholesterol, raised blood pressure, depression, sleep disorders, fatty liver, asthma, heart attacks, stroke, heartburn, reflux, incontinence, osteoarthritis and infertility. There's a good chance she won't live to an old age because of her weight.

If the life of a young woman is already in such turmoil, and the associated risks are so high, how could doctors not take her problem seriously? Maria was unable to go on, literally and figuratively, as if her life had been stranded like a ship on a sandbank.

Based on her weight and height, I calculated that she was over six stone overweight. She had gained that weight during her first pregnancy and had never managed to lose it again. She told me that she could no longer fit in a normal chair and that she struggled to wash herself properly. She looked pale, had an unpleasant body odour and very fine hair. She got out of breath tying up her shoelaces. She constantly tugged at her clothes, which kept getting stuck between her body's curves. Her children were also clearly overweight.

Maria asked whether her size could have anything to do with hormones. As a specialist in internal medicine, I always make a connection with hormone levels in cases like this. Patients don't generally do this, as the role of hormones in this field is less well known. Maria had already tried to lose weight many times and didn't know what to do. Most people would think: just eat less, and you'll lose weight. Your joints will be under less pressure and your pain will diminish. Move more too, and you'll automatically feel better and will have energy to socialise. Stop smoking, as that won't reduce stress but instead perpetuate it, and you'll save money too.

But that's all easier said than done. Maria couldn't afford the gym or a nutritionist, and vegetables cost more than frozen pizzas. Her attempts to stop smoking failed time and time again. Furthermore, she was gaining weight, and dragging an extra six stone around all day was bound to cause pain.

She was clearly consuming too many calories, but why? What was the real cause of her problem? Why had this woman got so big? And, more importantly, why was she staying so big?

She could answer this question easily herself: she was always hungry.

## Hunger and metabolism

Hunger is probably the oldest feeling on earth. We have been plagued with it for billions of years and people have tried all sorts of ways to take control of it. Hunger is more deeply entrenched in our bodies than feelings of love, awe and happiness; deeper even than other serious concerns like thirst, fear and shortness of breath. Satisfying hunger is vitally important to every animal. Extreme hunger leads to discrimination, war, murder and cannibalism. In the western world, we only know real hunger from the stories of those who experienced the Second World War and had to eat tulip bulbs, or from fairy tales in which hunger forces desperate parents to leave their children behind in the woods.

Every living thing on this earth, from single-celled organisms to thinking humans, is driven by the same urge to prevent a shortage of food. In humans, this takes place on all levels. Fundamentally, we are cells that each have their own metabolism and their own 'hunger'. This deep, basic metabolism can adapt to scarcity. Around it, layers have emerged that enable millions of cells to work together in a single body. In mammals, various cells became specialised and thereby formed separate systems – such as the digestive system – which are influenced, together with metabolism, by hunger and excess. All of these different cells communicate via our brain, which can influence virtually all our organs via the nervous system and hormones.

The brain enabled people to establish a food supply; agriculture and livestock farming were invented as a response to hunger, as was the food industry.

If we want to investigate how hunger works, we first need to look at the organs involved in metabolism. After that, we will discover how digestion and hormones are influenced by our metabolism, while the brain carries out its role as conductor, attempting to create a harmonious ensemble.

What happens within one cell, and therefore our bodies, is extremely complex. Building blocks – specifically amino acids, which are organic compounds that can be converted into other building blocks, such as proteins for muscles – are used to store energy in our bodies. This is known as metabolism, the process whereby the body alternately breaks substances down, processes them and stores them as energy. Ever since life existed, these cells have responded to a food supply. If a single-celled organism came into contact with a surplus of food, its metabolism led to the production of a surplus of substances that could be used for processes such as growth, repair or reproduction. If the cell didn't get enough food, however, the chemical reactions would stop. Any damage would no longer be repaired, the cell would be poisoned by its own waste products, and it wouldn't have enough energy to defend itself or multiply – essentially, a state of emergency.

This primordial cell will have perceived the scarcity as alarming, which is what still happens in every individual cell in our bodies today. If we encounter a shortage of food, all of our cells individually suffer from hunger. That's why real hunger can feel so overwhelming and all-encompassing. It is a deep and primitive feeling, and if it persists, everything – the whole body and the person themselves – is dominated by it and only one thing matters: finding food. That is not the same as having an appetite; it is a primitive drive for food, a genuine urge that can be felt in every cell in the body and is enough to make a person go crazy, but it can also cause serious defects because it causes bodily processes to stagnate.

For many of us in the modern, western world, our body's cells only experience real hunger under exceptional circumstances – if we suffer, for example, from a serious physical illness like anorexia. And in such cases, our body goes into survival mode on a cellular level – a function it has 'learned' over aeons of time through evolution. You might find it hard to believe that a single-celled organism can experience something like hunger but it can. It does register a change like a shortage of food and responds accordingly. Thanks to that powerful primitive impulse, species learned to adapt. Microorganisms that were able to store excess building blocks as reserves in times of abundance, and could switch to a power-saving mode in times of scarcity by keeping only the absolutely necessary processes running on a low setting, had a greater chance of survival.

This process represents an important mechanism for coping with hunger. In humans, this metabolic adaptation can take on extreme forms and can even have life-long consequences. Think, for example, of the women who were pregnant during the Dutch 'hunger winter' of 1944–45 (see Chapter 1), whose children had an increased risk of obesity and cardiovascular disorders. The scarcity these mothers experienced had a formative effect on the genes of their embryos, who were more likely to be overweight later in life. It was as if the mothers had passed on metabolic signals to prepare their children for a life of scarcity.

During puberty, the opposite can happen. The metabolism of young people (both men and women) who suffer from anorexia can remain in power-saving mode for life. The meagre energy the body possesses is reserved for those bodily processes that are strictly necessary and certain genes are definitively 'switched off' by substances released during extreme scarcity.[6] The genes, for example, that are responsible for feelings of hunger and satiety (such as the hormone leptin, which will be discussed in more detail later in this chapter) remain present in the DNA, but the cell is unable to make use of them.[7] This effect is called 'gene silencing' and is the opposite of hunger.

Whereas our metabolism is responsible for maintaining the energy balance of all our body's cells, digestion is the process of breaking down and absorbing the nutrients we obtain from our food. I will describe the role that hormones play in this ingenious system step-by-step.

## The stomach and our digestive system

Our digestive system is so important that its cells develop at a very early stage of life. In the first few weeks of a pregnancy, the embryonic endoderm is formed. This is where organs develop that are important for the intake of food: the digestive system (including gut, stomach, liver and gallbladder), the pancreas and the thyroid gland.

---

**Which organs and hormones are involved in digestion?**

**Mouth and salivary glands** (glandula parotis) – important for grinding food, producing saliva (enzymes that break down sugars) and helping control the quality of food.

---

**Oesophagus and stomach** (gastrum) – produce the hormones ghrelin and gastrin, which play a role in the digestion of proteins via gastric acid and the mixing of food.

**Liver** – produces bile (so that the fats in our diet can be digested and absorbed by the gut) and cholesterol (the building block for hormones).

**Small intestine** (duodenum) – produces cholecystokinin (CCK), serotonin and glucagon-like peptide (GLP-1), which are important for digestion (the absorption of sugars, fats and proteins) as well as intestinal function.

**Pancreas** – produces insulin and glucagon. Insulin regulates the blood sugar level and ensures that glucose is absorbed by your body. Glucagon increases the level of sugar in the blood. Both are important for fat metabolism.

**Abdominal fat tissue** (adipocytes) – produces leptin and oestradiol (from testosterone). Important for your energy reserves.

**Large intestine** (colon) – ferments sugars and fibres via gut bacteria and absorbs water from faecal matter.

The stomach is one of Mother Nature's fantastic inventions, designed to protect us from scarcity. But it can lead to obesity. In order to understand how that can happen, we first need to understand how digestion works.

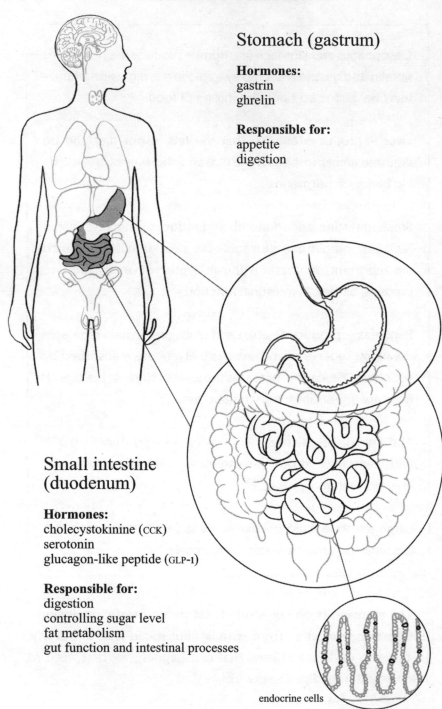

## Stomach (gastrum)

**Hormones:**
gastrin
ghrelin

**Responsible for:**
appetite
digestion

## Small intestine (duodenum)

**Hormones:**
cholecystokinine (CCK)
serotonin
glucagon-like peptide (GLP-1)

**Responsible for:**
digestion
controlling sugar level
fat metabolism
gut function and intestinal processes

endocrine cells

The first phase begins before we even start eating. Just thinking about, smelling or seeing food can be enough to make us salivate. The Russian physiologist Ivan Pavlov (see also the Introduction to this book) showed how this process works in animals as early as 1897.[8] In humans too, this reaction is triggered by the brain acknowledging that food is nearby. Glands in the mouth stimulate the release of saliva so that food can be swallowed more easily. Until Pavlov made his discovery, that slimy goo was certainly not a hot topic, but we now know that saliva contains all sorts of important hormones – a wealth of signalling substances! – including insulin and cortisol. Our brain also encourages the stomach to prepare itself for a meal. The release of gastrin stimulates the production of gastric acid, so that our food can be immediately digested once it arrives in the stomach.[9]

In the next phase, the presence of food causes the stomach to stretch slightly. This stretching is perceived by special receptors that send a signal to the brain via the nervous system. The brain, in turn, sends a signal back to the stomach to produce additional gastric acid. The food then moves to the small intestine. There, special cells detect the relatively acidic food mush from the stomach and subsequently release the hormones glucagon-like peptide (GLP-1) and cholecystokinin (CKK).[10] These hormones cause the pancreas and gallbladder to release digestive juices and enzymes; the digestive enzymes break down nutrients like sugars, fats and carbohydrates into small particles that can be absorbed into our bodies more easily. The liver and gallbladder subsequently release bile, which further aids the digestion of fats. Together, this makes the food mush less acidic and means that the digestive enzymes from the pancreas can do their work effectively.

The digested food is ultimately absorbed into the body's cells via the bloodstream with the help of insulin. There it forms the fuel

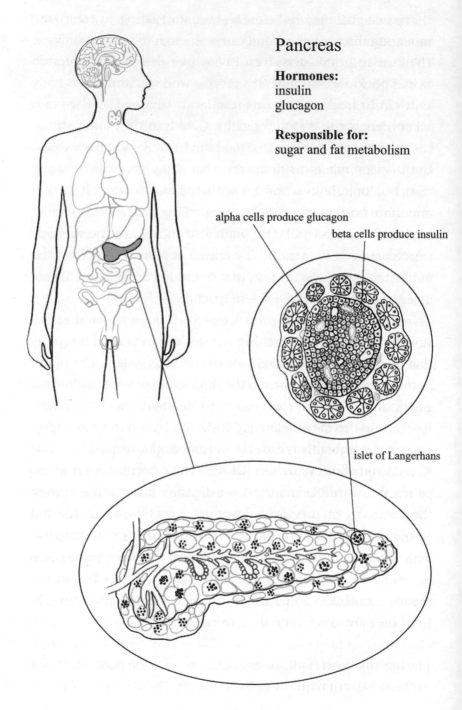

# Pancreas

**Hormones:**
insulin
glucagon

**Responsible for:**
sugar and fat metabolism

alpha cells produce glucagon

beta cells produce insulin

islet of Langerhans

that powers all the important bodily processes: from your heart rate and breathing, your hormone levels and digestive system, to repairing and restoring body cells and, of course, reproduction. In humans, the entire process of breaking-down food into nutrients, absorbing these substances and transporting them to all corners of the body, only takes a few hours.

The stomach's function is to delay feelings of hunger. I like to use the example of a lion to show how this works.[11] Driven by hunger, a lion hunts zebra. It might catch one or two a week: just enough to survive. If it didn't have a stomach, the zebra meat would be digested while the lion was still eating and it would immediately flow into the lion's bloodstream as amino acids. Within half an hour, the lion would be full. Hyenas and vultures would eat the rest of the prey and the lion wouldn't have enough energy to get through the following days. However, because the lion has a stomach, it can eat the entire zebra, because its hunger is not immediately satisfied while eating its prey.

It works the same way in humans. The stomach delays the digestion process and acts as a type of built-in lunchbox, in which you can safely carry your meal around without having to digest it immediately. The stomach itself adds some acid to it, a powerful preservative that ensures the food doesn't go off in the meantime. It is only digested when you are able to rest. The stomach then opens its sphincter and the food that has been mixed with the acid passes through to the small intestine. This process is controlled by hormones that act as a brake pedal (somatostatin) and as an accelerator (ghrelin).[12] These allow the stomach to delay digestion by around three hours in humans: long enough to search for more food in order to secure sufficient reserves to get through a period of hunger. This wonderful mechanism protected our distant ancestors from scarcity.

There are still many misunderstandings when it comes to the

stomach. It is not true, for example, that fatter people have bigger stomachs. You don't get fat from having a big stomach and eating a lot doesn't make your stomach any bigger. Your appetite doesn't depend on the size of your stomach either; an excessive appetite is probably the result of a faulty connection between hormone and nerve impulses from the stomach to the brain and vice versa (unless you have had surgery on the stomach, such as a gastric bypass, but we will return to that later in this chapter).

# Hunger makes small children big

Many parents are amazed by the sheer quantity of food their teenage children get through. They can eat whatever they want without gaining any weight, while their parents seem to gain weight just by looking at food. This not only shows how much energy the teenage years demand, but also how important metabolism is when it comes to maintaining a healthy weight. Hormones play a role here too. Both the satiety hormone leptin as well as the hunger hormone ghrelin are involved in the regulation of teenagers' appetites and the rate at which children grow during puberty.[13] This growth happens so quickly because their bodies convert carbohydrates, proteins and fats into usable forms of energy. A greater muscle mass and the ability to eat a lot without gaining weight are two of the side effects of puberty.

Unfortunately, there are also negative side effects of such a tightly adjusted hormonal balance. To put it simply, people tend to make decisions more quickly when they are hungry. This can have far-reaching consequences. Research has shown, for example, that hungry judges are more likely to make judgments to the detriment of the person on trial, and that these judgments would have gone the other way if they had been made after lunch.[14]

Incidentally, this knowledge is not new. In the sixth century AD, for example, judges in the Byzantine Empire were forbidden from making judgments unless they had eaten. A similar pattern is seen with doctors who have to decide whether or not to prescribe antibiotics: a full stomach results in a better-considered decision.[15] That's no different when it comes to adolescents.

During puberty, hunger hormones and satiety hormones therefore impact behaviour. This is one of the many ways your stomach is connected to your brain – a connection sometimes referred to as the gut-brain axis. Nerves run from the gut directly to the brain. By this pathway, but also via the release of hormones into the bloodstream, the gut gives signals to the brain. If you drink a few glasses of water before a meal, for example, you will eat considerably less.

This axis also plays a role after puberty. That's why it's not a good idea to go food shopping when you're hungry; you'll be much more likely to end up with a trolley full of food that is high in sugar and calories.[16]

## Modern lifestyle

In today's society, in which abundance is the norm, few people ever experience real hunger. On the contrary, a lack of exercise and an excess of high-calorie food leads to high levels of obesity. Three-and-a-half centuries ago, the Dutch doctor Steven Blankaart had great faith in sugar. In his *Borgelyke Tafel* (1683),[17] he describes his repeated observations of 'the disorderly way of eating that has crept in amongst certain prominent citizens' and how he believes sugar can neutralise the acid that makes our bodies sick, which is why its consumption is especially good for our physical well-being.

For a long time after crusaders brought the 'white gold' from Asia to Europe in the late Middle Ages, sugar was predominantly seen as something positive. It was a luxury product, which was available as a medicine in medieval pharmacies. In the 1970s, soft drinks were still marketed for babies and other high-sugar products were marketed for exhausted mothers. Today's scientists, however, never take anything as read; the fact that our amicable relationship with sugar has since cooled is vitally important for our heath. Since the 1970s, the composition of our diet has changed dramatically; products contain fewer nutrients and are combined with more sugars and preservatives, resulting in higher levels of obesity.

Besides not enough exercise and too much of the wrong types of food, our sleep is no longer what it once was; since the industrial revolution, the average person hasn't been getting enough sleep. In the west, we are sleeping an hour less per night than we were a hundred years ago, sleep guru Matthew Walker writes in his book *Why We Sleep*.[18] Our 24-hour economy means that almost one in five of the working population works evening and night shifts, which disrupts the circadian rhythm. This goes hand in hand with hormone fluctuations, including those responding to stress, or similar.[19] A major lack of judgement caused by disrupted sleep patterns may have played a role in the Challenger Space Shuttle disaster and the Chernobyl disaster, both in 1986.[20] Doctors are not immune to a lack of sleep either; they are more likely to make medical errors during night shifts.[21]

People who don't work night shifts can also experience disrupted sleep; approximately 30 per cent of all adults report sleep problems.[22] According to Matthew Walker, long-term exposure to artificial light, changed eating patterns (which means we often go to bed on a full stomach) and the time we spend on a phone, tablet or computer all contribute to disrupted sleep.

As a result, we are exposed to artificial light for longer, which impacts the production of melatonin, the hormone that makes us feel sleepy. Walker's advice is to avoid screens for an hour before bed.

Natural light also appears to have an effect on our sleep. A recent study showed that the average person sleeps twelve minutes less in summer than winter, and twenty-five minutes less in spring than winter.[23] That is probably due to the fact that we have almost four hours more daylight in spring and summer than in winter, and daylight has a positive effect on our biological clock.

Our sleep has deteriorated since the industrial revolution in terms of quality and quantity.[24] According to the American historian Roger Ekirch, people (like most animals) slept in two distinct phases until around two centuries ago. These phases, called the 'first' and 'second' sleep would each last around four hours, and the person would be awake in between. The French doctor Laurent Joubert (1529–82) is quoted in Ekirch's book *At Day's Close*[25] as advising people to have sex in this interim phase, as this was when people would experience greater pleasure and be able to perform better ... The biological basis of this biphasic sleep was partially unravelled in the 1990s by the American psychiatrist Thomas Wehr.[26] He showed that when healthy volunteers resided in an environment kept dark for fourteen hours each day, they too began displaying this biphasic sleep pattern – associated with the improved release of hormones such as melatonin and growth hormone – after a few weeks.

Although this sleep theory is viewed with scepticism, an increasing number of studies appear to confirm the link between a lack of sleep, working night shifts and the development of obesity and diabetes.[27] In short, the combination of how we are programmed and our modern lifestyle can easily lead to obesity due to disruption of the gut-brain axis. That excess weight and those poor sleeping and eating habits can cause people like Maria to end up in a vicious circle.

Should she therefore consider a gastric bypass?

## A balancing act: set-point weight

At the end of the last century, brain researchers discovered a receptor in the hypothalamus believed to be involved in the release of growth hormone. This hormone, which was previously unknown, is produced in the stomach and called ghrelin (growth hormone-releasing peptide).[28] We also encountered ghrelin in Chapter 3. It soon became clear that ghrelin doesn't actually have a lot to do with growth, but is mainly involved in maintaining a stable body weight.[29] In light of the west's growing obesity epidemic, research into this hormone is extremely relevant.

Ghrelin is produced by the empty stomach. The concentrations of the hormone in the blood are highest before a meal and lowest afterwards. It is therefore seen as a hunger hormone, whose role is to announce that the stomach is empty. We now know that men who are exposed to sunlight produce more ghrelin and consume more calories during the summer months. This isn't the case with women because of the preventative effect of oestrogens.[30] Ghrelin also influences the speed at which we make decisions,[31] especially in the centres of the brain related to addiction. It stimulates the brain to release dopamine, the feel-good chemical. As we want that pleasant feeling more often, we treat ourselves to something like a glass of wine or a bar of chocolate. That's how an addiction or dependency is formed and could perhaps explain why some obese people appear to have a genuine food addiction. Maria also mentioned that she ate more whenever she stopped smoking, as if the one addiction replaced the other. Recent research has shown that people are twice as likely to develop an alcohol addiction after having gastric bypass surgery.[32] And there are cases where an eating addiction is replaced by a gambling or sex addiction.

The interesting thing about ghrelin is that this hormone, which encourages people to eat, is present in higher concentrations in the blood of obese people than people of a healthy weight. Do obese people eat more because their stomach produces more ghrelin? Or is it the other way round: they are less sensitive to this hormone, so they need higher concentrations of it? It is difficult to say. Evidently, a system is active on a hormonal level that helps the body maintain a stable weight. If you want to stay fat, you will need to eat more. And that's where a stomach that produces more ghrelin comes in. At the same time, this doesn't sound logical: you might think – and want! – to be less hungry when you start getting too fat.

Our body seems to do all it can to maintain an increased weight by increasing its calorific requirement. It's as if we have a type of built-in thermostat that keeps our weight precisely at the right level: the set-point weight.[33] This explains the yo-yo effect we often see when people diet, whereby someone who has lost a lot of weight quickly puts it all – or sometimes even more – back on again.

Maria, who weighed over twenty stone at the age of thirty-five, is a prime example of this. The same effect is also seen in people who have gastric bypass surgery due to obesity; if such an operation needs to be reversed for whatever reason, the patient's weight will immediately increase and end up almost exactly the same as it was before the initial intervention, even if it was carried out years previously.

This set-point weight is controlled by the hypothalamus, the magic place deep in our brain that also ensures our body temperature remains stable. Contrary to our temperature, which fluctuates around 37 degrees Celsius throughout our lifetime, the set-point weight appears to be adjusted upwards over the years.[34] Those who eat more over a long period of time not only achieve a higher body weight, but also a higher set-point weight, making it harder to return to the previous weight. This set-point weight, maintained by ghrelin, means that your body weight has a tendency to continually increase (even when we don't want it to).[35] Unlike your salary, which you only ever want to increase, not fall!

In this way, ghrelin forms the perfect keystone for the business model of all fast-food chains. Sell your customers tasty burgers, but serve as much high-calorie food as possible on top for a small amount of money: soft drinks and fries! This small investment will make sure your customers gain weight. And if they eat high-calorie food for long enough, they will automatically develop a higher set-point weight and higher concentrations of ghrelin when their stomachs are empty. As a result, their need to keep eating your burgers will continually increase.

From the perspective of the obesity epidemic, ghrelin is a pointless hormone. Why would the body want to remain overweight? Excess weight leads to cardiovascular diseases, diabetes and knee problems. But from a biological point of view, it is in fact very useful. If an animal manages to live in a place of abundance, it will be successful. Its hunger will be satisfied, it will gain weight and its set-point weight will increase. Humans aren't any different in this respect. Our set-point weight will have been high at the start of humanity. As a result, our hunger had a powerful additional stimulus, which encouraged us to be inventive. We went out hunting for our food and, while searching for calories, populated the whole world.

Although ghrelin is clearly involved in weight, eating and hunger, the question is whether or not the term 'hunger hormone' is appropriate. This is because ghrelin is produced in other places too: the pancreas, the kidneys, the ovaries, the testicles and the lungs. And the opposite effect is seen in the event of gastric bypass surgery for obesity; although the stomach remains permanently empty after a gastric bypass, ghrelin concentrations decrease, rather than increase.[36]

The gene responsible for the production of ghrelin also works in a more complicated way than you might expect. Perhaps ghrelin and its growth hormone receptor did something a long time ago that was completely different from what we see them do today. Or is the evolution of the hunger hormone just as complex as that of hunger itself?

# The sum of energy

Let's return to Maria and ask ourselves why she is struggling to lose weight. Does her body not want to get rid of the weight she gained? That would only be part of the answer, because an adult's body weight is not simply the sum of mass, but also the result of energy.

A body gets that energy, expressed in calories, from nutrients. These are continually needed for metabolism, the musculoskeletal system and all other bodily processes. If you consume more than you use, your body stores all the excess calories in the form of mass: you gain weight. If you consume less than you use, your body turns to its reserves and you lose weight. If consumption and expenditure are the same, your body weight remains stable. That's simple maths. But it's not the case that 'eat less + move more' can solve everything. Unfortunately, it's not that straightforward.

A person with a higher body mass uses more energy. Their muscles also have to work harder to carry out the same movements due to that additional weight. An overweight person therefore has a higher total consumption of energy. So Maria not only has to eat more than normal to gain weight (the set-point weight), but also to remain overweight. Yes. In line with our knowledge about primordial cells, there are clear indications in the scientific literature that the human body is not inclined to get rid of excess fat tissue.

But my patient told me a different story. She felt that at a certain point in her life – after her first pregnancy – she had gained weight and had since been unable to lose it. Apart from the fact that you eat more as a pregnant woman, it may be the case that you change so much hormonally after a pregnancy (see Chapter 6) that your weight increases. A change to gut bacteria (again, see Chapter 6) could also play a role. You also require less energy as you get older because your muscle mass slowly decreases, and most people are less active after the age of twenty than they were in their youth due to work and family commitments. It's therefore quite possible that Maria's obesity was caused by an unfortunate combination of a changed eating pattern, hormonal changes, disturbances to her metabolism and a lack of exercise.

## The hormonal brake on obesity

As times of abundance were once rare, we as a species had to find ways to live with scarcity. That's why all organisms have numerous adaptations for securing as much food as possible – think of the giraffe's neck, the eagle's beak and the way ants work together – but hardly anything to protect us from excess.

Animals appear to be virtually insatiable. We use that to our

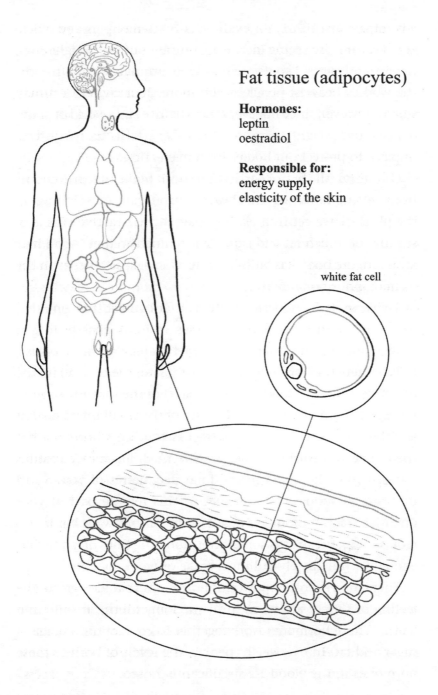

## Fat tissue (adipocytes)

**Hormones:**
leptin
oestradiol

**Responsible for:**
energy supply
elasticity of the skin

white fat cell

advantage; just think, for example, of fattened pigs and chickens. Vets are also seeing increasing numbers of overweight dogs, rabbits and cats.[37] People are insatiable animals too. Currently, the world's heaviest people weigh more than eighty or ninety stone. However, since not everyone who lives in a world of abundance is overweight, there are obviously certain control systems in place to protect our bodies from overeating.

Our mind (the brain) has an important brake that prevents us from getting fatter; we are always subconsciously weighing up the pleasure we get from eating against the negative effects of storing too much fat and gaining too much weight. At a lower level too, the body has built-in protection against obesity in the form of a hormonal brake.

There are two endocrine systems that control this: one that works in the short term and provides an immediate feeling of satiety, and another that affects satiety later, but more powerfully. Where the hormone ghrelin stimulates the body to fill the digestive tract with food at the very start of the process, another hormone is produced right at the end of the small intestine that lets the body know when this tract is full. This hormone has the rather uninspiring name, peptide YY 3-36, or PYY, and it's released into the blood in the final decimetres of your small intestine as soon as food arrives in this remote part of your digestive tract. It promotes digestion in various ways but it also reduces appetite. It says something along the lines of 'enough is enough', immediately pulling a brake on your appetite.

There are two other powerful hormones that also create the feeling of satiety after a meal in the longer term: insulin and leptin. These hormones work together to control the storage of sugar and fat. In overweight people, the levels of both of these hormones in the blood are significantly raised.

# Leptin

In 1949, a white mouse in a laboratory in the United States had offspring that couldn't stop eating. The mice ate themselves fat and passed this characteristic on to their offspring too. They had a congenital defect caused by faulty DNA. The mice were referred to as 'ob' mice, derived from the word 'obese'.[38] The inherited mutation in the DNA was located in the gene that produces a hormone that was only discovered half a century later: leptin (derived from the Ancient Greek *lepto*, which means 'thin'). This hormone is produced by fat cells and suppresses the compulsion to eat in the brain.[39] Usually, leptin protects mice from becoming overweight. If a mouse becomes too fat, it has more fat cells that produce more leptin, suppressing the compulsion to eat. As a result, it loses weight. However, because the ob mice didn't produce leptin as a result of the faulty gene, their compulsion to eat was not suppressed. As a result, they continued eating and got fat.

---

### Diabetes + insulin

The Danish Nobel Prize winner August Krogh had noticed that his wife, who had given birth to their fourth child a year previously, needed to urinate more often, had a decreased appetite and wasn't able to see as well as she used to. The married couple, both doctors, were quick to diagnose her with diabetes, but in 1921 the only treatment to reduce an elevated blood sugar level was a low-carbohydrate diet.

Thanks to his medical background, Krogh knew that the cause of this disease was the deficient production of

---

insulin by certain cells in the pancreas. These cells had been discovered by the German scientist Paul Langerhans in 1869. Because they looked like little clusters under the microscope, he named them the 'islets of Langerhans'. Fifty-two years later, the hormone was given the name 'insulin'. In 1890, Russian researchers had shown that dogs whose pancreases were surgically removed suffered from acute diabetes. Krogh had heard about a pair of young and ambitious doctors in Toronto called Frederick Banting and Charles Best who were able to isolate insulin from a dog's pancreas. When they readministered this insulin to the dog Marjorie (whose pancreas they had previously surgically removed), Banting and Best stabilised Marjorie's previously elevated blood sugar levels. Krogh decided to travel to Toronto and ask the doctors whether insulin could also be used on human patients with diabetes.

The pair found the answer in a slaughterhouse, where there were enough pancreases from freshly slaughtered calves to obtain the required insulin. Banting and Best were so pleased with their discovery that they granted Krogh a licence to produce insulin for the European market for just one dollar, on the condition that he would set up a non-profit company. This company, which ultimately became Novo Nordisk, would go on to become a global player in the field of diabetes medication.

This discovery was followed closely in the Netherlands too. The Dutch flagship company Organon was founded in the 1920s by Salomon 'Saal' van Zwanenberg with the help of the brilliant chemist Marius Tausk and the professor of pharmacology Ernst Laqueur, known as the founding father of endocrinology in the Netherlands.[40] Laqueur was one of the first to successfully produce hormone preparations from the glands and organs of slaughter cattle. Together they built a large international pharmaceutical company based on treatment with hormones like insulin, but also the thyroid hormone T4 and testosterone. They also helped develop the contraceptive pill (see also Chapter 7). A great-granddaughter of Laqueur wrote a wonderful novel about the origins of this factory.[41]

In humans too, mutations in the leptin gene can cause a child to have an innate, uncontrollable urge to eat. Taken as a medication, leptin helps these children get their weight under control, but the substance is difficult to create synthetically. There's also another, better-known hormone that is much more effective at controlling our metabolism (more about this in Chapter 6) and has extended the lives of hundreds of millions of people, albeit without the beneficial effects on weight: insulin.

All in all, the insatiability of metabolism may explain why a person can continue to eat too much and gain weight. The digestive system's hunger and satiety hormones show how efficiently they work and how the body evidently prefers being fat to thin. Being fat in times of abundance is no great feat. For most people, being seriously overweight leads to insulin resistance, which means the pancreas has to work overtime. Like a muscle, a gland can also tire and become depleted. And that's when type 2 diabetes arises, whereby insufficient insulin is produced. In that case, patients have to eventually resort to insulin injections. This type of treatment is especially onerous because patients have to inject themselves and because insulin causes additional weight gain.

Insulin is both a blessing and a curse.

## Hunger and the link between our gut and brain

The hormonal interplay between metabolism and digestion doesn't fully explain why Maria weighed twenty stone, while most people around her weren't as heavy. After all, they too lived in a society in which calories are continually imposed on them. In order to understand this, we need to take a closer look at the brain and nervous system.

We've seen that metabolism at a cellular level and the hormonally controlled digestive system influence the regulation of hunger and weight. Another factor is our brain – the biggest instigator of almost all bodily processes. Surprisingly, there are close links between the brain and the digestive tract, which has its own fascinating nervous system and is a similar size to our brain. It is with good reason that our gut is sometimes called our 'second brain'.[42]

It used to be said that if you weren't strong, you'd better be smart. But the brain itself uses vast amounts of energy. Fortunately, people had handy ways of consuming as many calories as possible. If you only pluck the ripe fruit, for example, you get more calories from less food because ripe fruit contains the most sugar. You can recognise ripe fruit from its sweet flavour and blue, red or dark-yellow colour. With an animal carcass, most nutrients and calories are found in the muscles and marrow, which contain an abundance of proteins and fats. These can be recognised from the fatty and salty flavour, and dark-red colour. In order to choose the best-quality, high-calorie parts when picking fruit or gutting an animal, our predecessors needed three things: a clever mind, skilled hands and good eyes. Humans are one of the few species of mammal with 3D colour vision, which allows us to perceive subtle differences in colour between ripe and high-quality, and unripe and rotten, from a distance.

The anatomical structure of our hands is also remarkably complex. We can hold something very precisely between our thumb and index finger in a pincer grip. This is extremely handy when it comes to sorting small objects, such as removing unripe and rotten berries from a pile, taking the rotting intestines out of a carcass, separating juicy leaves from hard ones, picking the most tender pieces of meat out from between the bones, digging the best roots out of the ground and peeling fruit. In order to process these 3D colour images, to make the right decisions and to then control the fine motor skills of two complex hands, a big brain is necessary: that's why we're called *Homo sapiens*, which means 'wise human'.

In the development of obesity, that marvellous brain unfortunately plays a detrimental role. And that is because of something interesting: the fact that people perceive high-calorie food as 'tasty'. If something tastes sweet or delectable, our brain rewards us for making the right choice with a pleasant sensation. In the animal kingdom, this phenomenon is relatively new. A hungry hyena eats a rotting zebra cadaver whole. It doesn't care whether or not it tastes good, as every bit of food helps satisfy its hunger. That wasn't the case for early Homo sapiens: they only enjoyed the most nutritious parts (meat, but also other food with high calorific values, such as fruit and grains), as that's how they would get most energy from each meal, which could then be stored in the fat tissue.

That new sensation of 'tastiness' has replaced the old sensation of 'hunger'. Humans didn't only seek food to satisfy hunger; they also sought tasty, high-calorie foods. That's how humans became selective omnivores, which was extremely beneficial to a small species that had struggled to hold its own around the large predators. With less physical effort, Homo sapiens were able to take in more food of a much higher quality, densely packed with calories and nutrients. As a result of their more efficient diet, they even had time left over to rest, daydream and fantasise, for example about the delicious berries and the mammoth they would find and catch the following day.

The first humans were social beings that lived and ate in groups. Children had a prominent position in society, as the group wouldn't have a future without them. As children couldn't eat as much as adults, they would get the best parts of the loot: those parts containing the most energy. This is how they learned from the adults, from a young age, what was high-quality and therefore tasty, and what wasn't. We still subconsciously teach our children to like sweet, red and flavourful food. It's not without reason that ketchup is so popular with children. It is as red as fresh meat and has an unmistakably rich flavour, but also contains more than 20 per cent pure sugar.

This is an important cause of today's obesity epidemic; people spoil their children by giving them the most delicious food. Whereas in the wild, the prehistoric man's metabolism would quickly convert high-quality and high-calorie food into energy for walking long distances and building houses, in today's world these are predominantly 'empty' calories that we eat purely because the food tastes good. This food acts as a filler as opposed to real nutrition, and our energy utilisation is completely different too. If sweets, crisps and ketchup had been available to the prehistoric man, we would have been too fat for thousands of years already.

Thanks to the brain, humans started making weapons and tools and discovered fire. This enabled them to cook, meaning they could consume food in easier, tastier ways. As a result, they turned their backs on hunting and gathering in order to develop new, hyper-selective ways of producing food: agriculture and livestock farming. One-sided food rapidly became more abundant. It was only a matter of time before something would go wrong.

## An ingenious brain results in complex eating behaviour

Our brain consists of various layers. For a basic function like 'eating', the metabolism, digestive system, hormones, nerves, muscles and brain are all involved. We have looked in detail at metabolism and the digestive system and have seen how a very complex interaction takes place in the outermost layer of our brain, the cerebral cortex, which results in our complex eating behaviour. This also explains the many types of psychological eating disorder that can lead to obesity, such as emotional eating, bulimia, stress eating and binge eating disorder.

Our behaviour is controlled not by a single layer of the brain, but by multiple layers (see the figure on page 120). The innermost layer of the brain, where the brainstem and hypothalamus are located, is called our 'first nature': our reptilian brain.[43] There we find the ancient instinct of human beings, the hunter-gatherers from whom we originate, who had to act fast in the event of danger. The vomeronasal organ, which was mentioned in Chapter 1, and pheromones also influence this innermost layer of the brain. That's why we want to consume anything that tastes good without constraint, our eyes are metaphorically bigger than our stomachs and we prefer to eat our food (after having smelled, tasted and felt whether it's good for us) alone or with our offspring. Mothers like to see their children eating well.

In humans, another layer formed around this innermost layer. This limbic system is called our 'second nature' and controls our emotional life. When humans gave up the freedom of hunting and gathering to become farmers, new rules of life were necessary. We now consider this set of morals self-explanatory; it is the cornerstone of our civilisation, comprising agreements about things like ownership and moderation. Whoever works (or inherits) most has access to the most food. Taking whatever was tasty became theft and waiting for the harvest became a virtue. The difference between poor and rich was expressed in a difference between fat and thin, as we saw with Princess Caroline and the miserable medieval Pope Innocent VIII.

In the outermost layer, our 'third nature' developed: the cerebral cortex, which houses our willpower and rationale. This comprises the rules of life for humans who no longer hunt, gather or cultivate. These are the societal rules and regulations, the religious food regulations, the governmental food guidelines, the food pyramid guide, the advice from the doctor, the diets. The 'third nature' bombards us with warnings that contradict our 'first nature': avoid carbohydrates, sugar and fat, don't overeat, don't skip breakfast, keep an eye on your cholesterol, count your calories, weigh your ingredients, use a food tracker app. People are even willing to pay for diets that will help them eat less. To the primitive man, this would have sounded completely bonkers!

The warnings or signals originate in our brain, a type of supercomputer that is also powered by electricity. The transmission of signals by the nerve cells takes place via electrical impulses. However, the actual transfer of an impulse from one nerve cell to another doesn't happen via electrical impulses, but via chemical substances called neurotransmitters.

An important neurotransmitter in the brain is serotonin, which we are familiar with from the feeling of being in love or having butterflies in our stomach. The substance not only affects our mood, but also indirectly affects our weight. We know this because many antidepressants also increase appetite and cause weight gain due to their effect on serotonin. Serotonin, mood and appetite are all connected.

More than 90 per cent of all serotonin in the body is made in the small intestine and potentially controlled by the bacteria that live there, but it's not yet clear exactly how serotonin influences the brain. There are indications that microbes in the gut play a role in weight gain, and that the residents of your gut influence not only appetite, but also mood. I will discuss this in more detail in Chapter 6.

## Is a gastric bypass a good idea?

Let's return to the question: should Maria have a gastric bypass in order to get rid of her excess weight? Despite her lack of exercise, she needs to consume an average of two thousand four hundred calories a day in order to maintain her current weight, the way her body wants it. In her case, a congenital defect relating to the production of the hormone leptin is not likely, as she only became overweight after her pregnancies. However, the high concentration of the hormone ghrelin in her blood will stimulate her sense of hunger. This, in the context of set-point weight, may explain why Maria feels so much hungrier than the people around her now that she has become overweight. And the cause may therefore relate to an epigenetic change: because she ate too much over a long period of time, this high food intake has been 'imprinted' in her genetic material.

But that's no reason to simply accept things the way they

are. This woman, like everyone else, has a powerful mechanism she can use to combat the weight that is impairing her life: her brain. With her brain, she can choose what she does and doesn't eat. However, that is precisely her problem. Those choices are what led to her gaining so much weight in the first place, either consciously or subconsciously. If she had lived in the prehistoric period, she would have become a successful hunter-gatherer, with successful children whom she would have taught to make the same choices. The scarcity of food would have kept her calorie intake in check (the reason why our predecessors weren't overweight, whereas obesity is prevalent today). Her problem is that she is making old choices in a new earthly paradise. The calories are there for the taking – even, or perhaps especially – for those who don't have much money.

One of the newer treatment methods for obesity is to administer a high dosage of the synthetic gut hormone GLP-1 in order to decrease the sense of hunger. The question around this is: how long does that effect last?[44] A bariatric operation on the digestive tract is much more invasive than daily injections with GLP-1, but by artificially restricting calorie intake and recalibrating the metabolism, the procedure can restore the balance.

Operations to tackle obesity are as old as the Roman Empire. Pliny the Elder dedicates a chapter to a fat young man in his *Natural History* (78 AD): 'It is also on record that the son of the consular Lucius Apronius had his fat removed by an operation and relieved his body of unmanageable weight.' The historian also claims that fat tissue is insensitive and does not contain any blood vessels.[45] It is likely that this operation was performed from time to time in the Roman Empire; a hundred years later a similar operation was described in the Talmud, with reference to the exceptionally fat rabbi Eleazar ben

Simon from Judea: 'And he was given a sleeping potion and taken to a marble room where his stomach was cut open and baskets upon baskets of fat were removed from it.'[46] The reason for the operation was both cosmetic as well as functional, 'as the good man apparently suffered from the size of his belly in the marital bed'.

It seems unlikely that the abdominal cavity itself was actually cut open in these operations, as Hippocrates had already known centuries earlier that this would be fatal and both men lived for years after their operations. In the case of the son of Lucius Apronius, it was probably not fat tissue that was removed, but excess skin. Apronius had been sent on a mission to Africa, where he probably lost a considerable amount of weight. In that case, the intervention didn't involve the removal of fat, but was instead what's now known as a tummy tuck, or abdominoplasty. This technique came into fashion in the 1960s after Ivo Pitanguy, a Brazilian surgeon, performed it on the American actress Elizabeth Taylor.[47] In the 1980s, the French surgeon Yves-Gérard Illouz came up with the brilliant idea of suctioning the subcutaneous fat away with a vacuum as opposed to cutting it out. With that, liposuction was invented. We now know that removing subcutaneous fat has a cosmetic effect, but doesn't do much to help the metabolism, which was the whole point of the procedure.

Other interventions that target the abdominal cavity appear to be more effective in terms of helping people lose weight. In the 1960s, the American surgeon Edward Mason experimented with stomach-reducing operations, with varying levels of success. In his scientific publication from 1969, he claimed that if the patient lost weight, it was as a result of Mason's surgery; if not, it was the patient's fault. He later refined the procedure to what is today's gold standard: a gastric bypass performed using keyhole (laparoscopic) surgery. As a result of this procedure, patients can expect to weigh a quarter less for the rest of their lives.[48]

Bariatric surgery (commonly referred to as 'gastric bypass') has greatly increased in importance in western society over the last twenty years, and is now the most common stomach operation in the world to combat obesity. At first glance, this weight-loss intervention might seem too easy a fix for a problem that someone has 'done to themselves'. But whatever you think, a gastric bypass operation that leads to improved hormone levels is currently the only treatment with a sufficiently sustainable result. The positive side effects of these operations also speak for themselves. Three quarters of patients with diabetes no longer require medication; the same number experience improvements to their health for the rest of their lives, giving them back the chance to age healthily.[49] Of course, the fact remains that an operation on the stomach doesn't address the root cause of the problem. But is this important if you can treat the effects? You might say: throw the ballast overboard, so the boat is free and can sail again. Remove the excess weight, and the patient can start living their life again.

In a gastric bypass, the intestine is connected to the top of the stomach, so the food passes directly to the intestine after swallowing it, where it can be digested. The food is therefore not subject to the three-hour wait in the stomach. This means that hunger can dissipate while the patient is still eating, but the patient will have to eat multiple small meals a day for the rest of their life.

This is the treatment that Maria received, and her operation was a success. She lost her extra six stone and hasn't put the weight back on again so far.

The gastric bypass, which is the last resort in the case of morbid obesity, also reduces the ability to perceive sweet flavours. As expected, a decreased desire for sweet things because of a change to our digestive hormones after the intervention contributes to weight loss, and vice versa: a less accurate perception of flavours can lead to weight gain if the body accidentally fails to send signals of satiety to the brain. The discrepancy between what we are tasting and what we are actually eating deceives the body when it comes to estimating the reserves in our cellular store cupboard.

Although the operation is remarkably safe and can be performed in less than an hour, the number of people with obesity or morbid obesity who would qualify for it has become so great that all the surgeons in the world wouldn't be able to operate on all of them, even if that was all they did for the rest of their lives. Gastric bypass surgery is therefore not the solution to the obesity epidemic. Obesity is an important risk factor for what we refer to as 'diseases of affluence': diabetes, cardiovascular disease and cancer. Morbidly obese people therefore have a shorter life expectancy. And this is the case all over the world; while infectious diseases and malnutrition were still the major causes of death in Africa until recently, these diseases of affluence are now increasing there too.

Perhaps the obesity epidemic will lead to a division of our species, and in the future we will speak of a *Homo sapiens proprius*, the true, healthy human with a long life expectancy, and the *Homo sapiens obesitate*, the human with obesity. This is precisely why it is important that when combating the obesity epidemic, we utilise our knowledge about hormones and their influence on our eating habits. By analysing this knowledge, we can develop new medicines and treatments. It's not yet clear whether the best way to do so is to supplement lacking hormones or to surgically intervene in the anatomy of the stomach, thereby indirectly affecting the mutual interplay between the brain, metabolism and digestive system.

Perhaps our gut bacteria also play an important role in the treatment of obesity ...

# 6

# Residents of Your Gut

*Key Players in Your Hormone Balance*

In autumn 2006, I was training as a doctor in internal medicine at Amsterdam University Medical Center. A melancholy patient in her eighties had been in our department for many months; she had developed chronic diarrhoea from a course of antibiotics used to treat a urine infection. Medication was no longer able to help. The diarrhoea was the result of an infection caused by the bacterium *Clostridium difficile*, which damages the intestinal lining and leads to severe abdominal pain, fever and cramps. Patients suffer from bouts of watery diarrhoea up to ten times a day, causing them to lose weight and become so weak that they end up completely bedridden.

Twenty per cent of patients with this infection ultimately succumb to it. It's therefore hardly surprising that many of them feel melancholy. As the woman had been lying in bed in a depressed state for so long, she was completely emaciated and had bedsores all over her body. It was a very grave situation.

# The Power of Hormones

The woman wanted nothing more than to go home to be with her husband, who had metastatic cancer. I could understand that only too well, and so off I went, perhaps overconfidently, in search of a treatment that would provide a short-term solution. My efforts were in vain, until I remembered a presentation from a conference a few years earlier, in which Johannes Aas, a gastroenterologist, had explained how he had treated such cases using the faeces of a healthy person after having read a publication about it from 1958.[1] By infusing healthy faeces with other bacteria, the proliferation of this troublesome bacterium is slowed down.[2] As a result, there is a battle between the bacteria, whereby the healthy type – which is best at multiplying – wins and ousts the bad Clostridium bacterium from the gut. What happens on a daily basis in nature can be supported in a body by means of a faecal transplantation. Only years after the presentation by the Norwegian doctor did the importance of his words become clear to me.

Within a week, after gaining the patient's consent, I had everything I needed ready for the first faecal transplantation in the Netherlands. I would have never thought you could use a simple food processor to prepare a stool solution ... One Friday afternoon we carried out the treatment by introducing stool obtained from the patient's son via colonoscopy. I sensed the excitement rising in the treatment room as everyone present, nurses and doctors alike, felt that something very special was about to happen.

The patient was safely returned to her room in the hospital that afternoon and, at first, nothing seemed any different. However, when I saw her after the weekend, it turned out that her chronic diarrhoea had, in fact, improved. The woman had been for a little walk for the first time in months and was in great spirits. She didn't have any side effects from the treatment, except that her melancholia had left without trace. She returned home the very next day, together with her husband. Thanks to the treatment, they were able to enjoy life together for several more years.

In 2014 *Gut* was published, written by Giulia Enders, a PhD student at Goethe University in Frankfurt, who was twenty-four at the time.[3] The book changed the impression that many readers had of their digestive system overnight. More than a million copies were sold in its first year of publication and it has since been translated into forty languages. *Gut* does away with the notion that the gastrointestinal tract is nothing more than a channel into which food and drink enter at one end and out of which faeces and farts exit at the other. Enders shows how complex and fascinating our gut is. And although this subject is more complicated than she would have us believe, I – as a researcher into the role of gut bacteria in endocrinological processes – completely agree with her on a number of points.

What has this got to do with our hormones? A lot. This is because the bacteria in our gut are indispensable when it comes to maintaining a healthy hormonal balance. They are involved in the release and production of dozens of different hormones.[4] Gut bacteria influence the creation of hormones and the function of the brain via the central nervous system.[5] Furthermore, bacteria in general often lead to the discovery of new medicines, ranging from antibiotics to cholesterol-reducing drugs.[6] In summary, the bacteria in and around us are key to a healthy life!

This chapter is all about the gut and its residents. What do we know about them and why does this subject belong in a book about hormones? And, more importantly, what can we do in order to maintain the right balance between our gut bacteria and hormones?

## Perhaps Hippocrates had the right idea all along

What we knew about the gut before the publication of *Gut* was the following: as your food travels through your gut, nutrients are removed and absorbed into the bloodstream through the intestinal wall. For those interested in the specifics of this process, here are a few details: the breakdown of starch begins in your mouth while you are still chewing. In the process, the first digestive enzyme, ptyalin, is released, which – like its sister amylase in the pancreas – breaks down starch from our food into carbohydrates.[7] Ptyalin is deactivated by the stomach acid it encounters when the food pulp arrives in your stomach. As the enzymes from your saliva were thoroughly mixed together with the food pulp while you were chewing the food, the digestion of carbohydrates continues for at least an hour, i.e. also in your small intestine, where the food arrives after passing through your stomach. That's why it is so important for your digestion to chew your food properly.

The proteins have already become smaller due to the acid in your stomach; now the enzyme pepsin further breaks down the proteins into amino acids, which in turn initiate the production of hormones in the gut. In the small intestine, the breakdown of carbohydrates into sugar (glucose) is then completed with the help of enzymes from the pancreas. Further on in the gut, fats are broken down into fatty acids so they can be burned more easily. Once your food has been thoroughly broken down into tiny pieces, these pieces are absorbed into the bloodstream through the intestinal wall via the lymph (the fluid that consists of white blood cells). The parts that remain, such as indigestible fibres, continue their journey and are combined with other waste products. In the final part of the gut, the large intestine, the remaining moisture, which contains a number of essential vitamins and minerals, is removed with the help of the digestive hormone GLP-1.[8] At the last part of the large intestine – the rectum – the waste materials leave our body and disappear down the toilet.

That is a brief version of the classic summary of our digestive system the way we learned it at school and the way it has been taught to medical students at universities for many decades.

However, according to Giulia Enders, our gastrointestinal tract is a much more complicated and also more ambitious organ. Our gut and its residents are responsible for the production of numerous different hormones and who knows how many other unknown hormone-like substances. I have already described the most important hormones involved in digestion: insulin, GLP-1 and CCK. Serotonin (produced in the small and large intestine) can also be added to the list.[9] Gut bacteria are important for our bowel movements and we now know that they are involved in the production of cortisol and adrenaline in the adrenal gland, and that pheromones are also produced in our faeces.[10] In summary, our gut is so much more than the producer of faeces and farts. You could even refer to it, in Enders' words, as an 'elegant ballet dancer'.

Her debut came at just the right time. Over the past fifteen years, our understanding of the true nature and function of the gut has fundamentally changed. Where in the past we could only study gut bacteria per culture using cultivation methods, we can now find out what's residing in our gut within a couple of hours by reading the genetic codes (DNA sequencing).[11] Some researchers over the past decades[12] have even gone as far as describing the gut as our second brain due to its influence on our behaviour – after all, your gut communicates with your brain via the nervous system and hormones.

We have actually already known that for some time. Expressions like, 'I've got a lump in my throat' and, 'My stomach is in knots' show that the connection between gut and brain is nothing new. We can be grateful to Giulia Enders for the fact that she has made the gut a bit more popular for a lot of people.

But there is a lot more to be said about this clever organ. Not only do we have a better understanding of how our gut works, but these new insights also contribute to what we know about our hormonal balance. Our well-being appears to depend greatly on our gut bacteria, for instance. A healthy gut not only provides resistance, but also gives us energy and higher levels of concentration. The residents of our gut determine whether we can remember lists of French vocabulary, whether we sleep well, how much and what we eat, and even how the emotional bond with our children is regulated in our brain.

However, besides all of these positive characteristics of gut bacteria, there are also bad bacteria that can negatively impact our body and how we function.[13] The University of Cambridge Professor of psychiatry Edward Bullmore wrote *The Inflamed Mind* in 2018. In this bestseller, he explains how a digestive system with bad gut bacteria can lead to illnesses like depression (through a lack of serotonin), Parkinson's disease (through a lack of dopamine) and dementia (through chronic inflammation of certain brain cells).[14] Hippocrates, the father of modern medicine, committed this same thought to paper 2,500 years ago: 'All disease begins in the gut.'

# Why we don't always hear about new insights

The complexity of our gut was written about long before Giulia Enders arrived on the scene. Joshua Lederberg, the American molecular biologist who won the Nobel Prize for Physiology of Medicine in 1958 at the age of thirty-three, proved to be a visionary.[15] Several decades ago, he recognised that a better understanding of the intestinal flora – and the production of pheromones and hormone-like substances that takes place in the gut – could contribute to a better understanding of how our body works. In 2001, he introduced the term 'microbiome': the collective name for the millions of microorganisms that are found in our gut, comprising bacteria, fungi, viruses and yeasts. They keep our gut healthy and protect us against germs. This insight led to a real revolution in biomedical science. But Lederberg still wasn't the first to recognise the importance of the intestinal flora. In books on Chinese medicine from the fourth century BC, the alchemist Ge Hong recommended a suspension made from the faeces of babies ('yellow soup') to treat depression and stomach complaints.[16] At the start of the last century, the British army officer and writer Thomas Edward Lawrence, better known as Lawrence of Arabia, was given tea made from camel faeces as a welcome drink by the Bedouins on the Arabian Peninsula. It was said that this would prevent illness. It is only in the past few years that this has been exposed as a myth.[17]

It sometimes takes a while to hear about new insights, even if they are actually already old, and it wasn't until the start of the twenty-first century that doctors recognised the practical benefits that the new term microbiome could entail, such as manipulation of the immune system and improvements to our metabolism and digestion. New knowledge often raises new questions: which gut bacteria are actually found in the gut and where exactly are they located? What do they do there? How do they get there? And – an important question in the field of medicine – how can we gain health benefits by influencing the intestinal flora?

Over the past ten years, research into the gut has exploded. The number of publications about the subject has increased seven-fold over the past five years (from 1,178 scientific articles in 2010 to 8,986 in 2021). This is thanks to the way in which the composition of gut bacteria can now be studied. A few years ago, a special science magazine (*Microbiome*) was launched that focuses on research into the composition and function of gut bacteria in humans and animals. Special microbiome conferences are held all over the world, the topic brings in venture capital, and start-up companies are springing up that want to benefit from the opportunities. Representatives of patient associations and big pharmaceutical companies are also stirring; everyone wants to play a part and get a share of the many opportunities the microbiome offers. These range from better diagnostics to new treatment possibilities. It remains to be seen whether these hopes will be fulfilled or if it is all just hype and hot air. But what does this microbiome mean in terms of improvements to our health? And how can scientists prove that bacteria are actually the cause of certain hormonal diseases?

## The residents of our gut

In 2002, I was on placement in the ear, nose and throat department at the Charité hospital in Berlin. I was assigned to a professor who had trained as a doctor in East Germany. The first time I met her, she told me, 'A good trainee doctor doesn't ask, but listens.' So, while I sat beside her on a stool in silence,

I became acquainted with all the infections that present themselves in the head and throat region.

That's where I came under the spell of Robert Koch (1843–1910) and his research into the influence of bacteria on the development of infections. Koch was a district doctor in Wolsztyn in Poland (Prussia at the time) and became fascinated in the saliva, stool and wound exudate of his patients – especially after his wife gave him a microscope as a birthday present. In a small corner of his surgery, he worked on one of the biggest discoveries in the world of medicine, which was deservedly awarded the Nobel Prize in 1905. What did he discover? That bacteria can cause infections.

After Koch started work as a professor in the Charité hospital (and walked the same corridors that I would walk almost a hundred years later), he published his 'Koch's postulates'.[18] These are a number of rules of thumb that doctors and scientists can use to establish whether certain bacteria and viruses cause human diseases. According to his criteria – as we saw with the COVID-19 pandemic – a bacterium or virus (or pathogen) must first be encountered in large numbers in a person. Secondly, it must then be possible for the pathogen to be isolated and cultured. Thirdly, after exposing a laboratory animal to the pathogen, it must cause the suspected disease (and the animal must be able to be cured again after treatment). Finally, the bacterium from the experiment with the animal must be the same as the one encountered with the patient.

The question remains: how can bacteria be transferred from one human to another in order to strengthen the effect of our hormones?

After successfully performing the first Dutch faecal transplantation at Amsterdam University Medical Center in 2006, the treatment was carried out on a similar group of patients in a large-scale study with equal success.[19] Since then, it has been included in the arsenal of treatments for the chronic diarrhoea associated with *Clostridium difficile* all over the world. As an endocrinologist, I became increasingly interested in the effects of donor faecal transplantations on the hormonal balance. We discovered, for example – this was later confirmed by further research – that a change to the gut bacteria composition makes a body more sensitive to *insulin*[20] and that the effect of serotonin and dopamine decreases in the brains of overweight people.[21] Consider, for example, how a lack of serotonin immediately makes people feel gloomy. Sterile mice that have never had a bacterium in their gut are more anxious than mice found in the wild, and less able to learn new things. Their digestive tract is also less well-developed.[22] To me, this seemed a good reason to take a closer look at the 'good' residents our guts are hosting and the 'squatters' we ought to be aware of.

In our bodies, bacteria generally group together in complex communities – referred to by Lederberg as 'microbiota' – most of which are found in the gut. Until fifteen years ago, it was only possible to see which bacteria were on the skin or in the stool by growing a bacterial culture. The organ, stool or liquid under investigation would be swabbed and then rubbed around a 'nutritious' plate (containing sheep's blood) a few times to reveal which bacteria were growing.

That was a difficult undertaking, because if there were not quite enough bacteria on the swab or if the bacteria didn't thrive when exposed to air, for example, nothing would grow. It's easy to see how this selective method led to a vast underestimation of the number of bacteria in the gut. Back then, it was assumed that only approximately three hundred types of bacteria lived in the gut. Since then, major progress has been made in terms of determining the exact composition of our gut. This is possible thanks to high-throughput screening for analysing bacterial DNA. This state-of-the-art technology has allowed us to establish that every gram of stool in a healthy gut contains thousands of different types of bacteria. That's considerably more than the three hundred types previously assumed to live there – and that's before taking viruses and fungi into account. What's more, these residents of the gut also release chemicals from our food. It was recently established, for example, that a volume of alcohol is produced in our gut each day that is equivalent to two to three bottles of beer in a healthy person and up to half a litre of whisky in an obese person.[23] Who would have thought we are running a small brewery in our belly!

So, there are many types of bacteria and they also have a far-reaching impact. The magician's box that the population of bacteria in our gut constitutes proves much more versatile than the once-held notion of a simple digestive tract. You could think of the gut microbiome (including fungi and viruses as well as bacteria) as an organ weighing roughly two kilograms that fulfils many different functions. As mentioned, it produces desirable hormones such as serotonin and dopamine, important for our mood, but it also generates harmful substances, such as the hormone-like substance kynurenine, made from tryptophan.[24] Elevated levels of this substance are found in the blood of patients with inflammatory bowel disease and can cause low mood and fatty liver. We also recently discovered that the immune cells from our bone marrow first travel to the small intestine, where they learn to differentiate between good and bad bacteria – a type of primary education for our immune system – before fulfilling their role as our body's defence system.[25] This 'training' sometimes goes wrong, causing the immune cells to turn against our hormone factory, which can result in an exhausted thyroid gland.[26]

Simply put, your gut bacteria are vital. In addition to taking care of the immune system, they also take as much energy as possible from your food – that is, if it stays in your gut long enough.[27] Due to a poorer composition of gut bacteria, people who are overweight have slower bowels (the transit time).[28] With mice, the composition of gut bacteria even affects body temperature and metabolism.[29] Since a diverse microbiome contributes to a better quality of sleep,[30] jetlag can shake up our internal residents in such a way that it disrupts the release of the sleep hormone melatonin.[31] It goes without saying that your metabolism is then affected too.

But what about the 'squatters', those bad bacteria you would rather not have in your own four walls? Don't forget that you have a built-in alarm – your immune system – which keeps intruders out. Your gut bacteria also work together to successfully ward off pathogens. If, for example, a bacterium that is resistant to antibiotics threatens to get the upper hand, the healthy intestinal flora responds immediately by providing extra protection to the intestinal lining.[32] The new resident is 'taken hostage' and a large-scale squatter movement cannot be formed.

Gut bacteria also work together by producing natural toxins to inhibit the growth of other bacteria. The best-known example of this type of toxin is penicillin, which – like almost all other antibiotics – provides one group of bacteria with a weapon by which to eliminate another group of bacteria. Bacteria can make bacteriocins, which destroy the bad bacteria in our gut,including those able to sustain a chronic stress reaction in our body.[33,34] In this way, the human body and gut bacteria have a mutually beneficial relationship.

# How do we end up with all those gut bacteria?

During pregnancy, the mother's gut bacteria change, probably under the influence of pregnancy hormones.[35] In the first and third trimester, the gut bacteria of an expectant mother are most similar to those of an overweight person, probably so the mother's gut can absorb as much energy as possible from food, giving the baby the best possible start in life. The way in which a child comes into the world also appears to play an important role in the development of their intestinal flora and the development of potential diseases at a later age. If the mother has a vaginal birth, bacteria from her gut are transferred into the baby's mouth and end up in the baby's gut. These bacteria are presented to the newborn baby's defence system via both the vagina and the bloodstream, which stimulates and nurtures the baby's immune system so that it can better respond to any unknown bacteria it encounters.

It therefore appears that bacteria from the gut are more diverse and more 'pathogenic' than bacteria from the mother's skin. A child born by caesarean section is placed against the mother's skin and, in that case, the skin bacteria will enter and populate the gut via breastfeeding. This does, however, make a big difference. The skin bacteria are received by the gut's immune system in a friendlier way, which means they can multiply more easily there. At the same time, the child's immune system is less well 'trained' as a result. It is an easier dance – not a tango, as Giulia Enders would say – and a consequence of this is the immune system struggles to master the difficult steps.

This can cause problems at a later age. If you have never learned to deal with these unknown bacteria, pathogens (for example after food poisoning) are more likely to enter your microbiome. They can then take hold and cause great damage – for example, by causing immune disease of the thyroid and pancreas[36] – whereas what we want is for these harmful bacteria to have no chance there. Fortunately, it is possible to 'train' caesarean section babies. Katri Korpela, a researcher in the field of the microbiome at the University of Helsinki, recently led a study in which babies born via caesarean section were treated with a suspension containing their mother's faeces by means of a mini faecal transplantation. Through her study, Korpela demonstrated that babies have a much healthier start in life if the mother's vaginal and gut bacteria (as opposed to skin bacteria) are able to take hold in the newborn's gut.[37]

Whether or not you are born by caesarean section, your intestinal flora develops from birth onwards into a complex and stable community of microorganisms. Viruses, fungi, parasites and bacteria live – if all is well – harmoniously together. If one of the residents takes up too much space, this is rectified by the other gut bacteria and their hormone-like substances, as previously mentioned.

The development of such a community has its ups and downs, and the environment in which the baby is raised also plays a role. In the past, it was completely normal for a baby to be breastfed by various women. Recent research shows that whether or not a baby is breastfed has a big influence on the formation of favourable (or unfavourable) strains of bacteria in the baby's gut, as the immune system is either better or less well adjusted, which influences the likelihood of disease later in life.[38]

## Poop group!

Interestingly, we have discovered that cohabiting family members share microbiota with each other. It even appears that people share up to 50 per cent of their microbiota with their pets.[39] People can be divided into groups on the basis of a certain composition of their gut bacteria, the way we do with blood types. These so-called 'enterotypes' or 'poop groups' are not related to nationality, sex, age or weight, but diet is an important common factor.[40] What's striking is that these poop groups can also influence the effect of thyroid hormone and insulin.[41,42]

Before long, hospitals may be able to offer tests to determine our poop group. This would then help us detect certain (endocrine) disorders at an earlier stage. Our gut microbiome not only contributes to our general well-being, but may also shed light on our susceptibility to certain diseases, or the effect of a diet, the consequences of alcohol consumption and possibly even the effects of medication. It may well be the case that paracetamol is less effective for person A who went out last night and woke up with an awful hangover than for person B, who also drank too much but, due to their genes, has more bacteria in their gut that don't break down the components of paracetamol before they are absorbed into their bloodstream. Of course, these are only hypotheses, but there is no doubt whatsoever that further research in this field is called for.

## What the future might hold for us

In the same way that a healthy gut microbiome keeps you fit, changes to its composition can lead to endocrine disorders. And even though a lot of research is needed before we can understand exactly how that works, there are already important insights that may be able to help us. According to Professor Martin Blaser, doctor and microbiologist at Rutgers University in New Jersey, the diversity of our intestinal flora can decrease so drastically due to the frequent use of antibiotics and our western lifestyle that it can often take months before it recovers – and in many cases it never manages to fully regain a balance.[43] We recently discovered that the intestinal flora of indigenous people of the Amazon, who have never taken antibiotics or consumed a western diet, is 30 per cent richer than ours.[44] An interesting detail is that there is virtually no diabetes and obesity in this population. Based on the fact that 50 per cent of your intestinal flora comes from your parents and the other 50 per cent from your environment, Blaser believes there will be a loss of diversity of gut bacteria with every new generation.[45] With this information in mind, take another look, without prejudice, at your child's full nappy.

Is there any hope for people with a 'poor' gut bacteria composition? As mentioned, donor faecal transplantations are already available in hospitals and are able to improve the composition of your intestinal flora, at least temporarily. They are currently available as elegant capsules – somewhat more appealing than eating faeces – and some private clinics already offer this type of treatment for big sums of money.[46] Although I think it is still too soon for commercial treatments with faecal transplantation, further research could offer insights into the hormonal treasure chest our gut bacteria are likely to constitute for our health. The significance of this new knowledge for the individual patient remains to be seen.

It's sometimes useful to look back on what was written thousands of years ago. Doctors have known for some time that the thyroid, which acts as our body's metronome by aligning heart rate, temperature and metabolism, plays an important role in metabolism. It has been known for thousands of years that our gut stops working effectively in the event of a lack of thyroid hormone. That is perhaps why the Greek surgeon and pharmacologist Dioscorides, who lived in the first century after Christ and wrote the pharmacopoeia *De materia medica*, worked on an early version of faecal transplantation. He tried desperately to help thyroid patients by administering them the faeces of healthy dogs and lizards.[47] Although his book doesn't explain why he chose these species in particular, he was obviously well-acquainted with the relationship between normal stool and an effective thyroid function.

While faeces were, for many years, seen as the useless and malodorous end product of metabolism, it now seems to be becoming a new treatment method. Just think, for example, of consuming of a bacterial strain drink designed especially for you to prevent you from developing rheumatism or diabetes, or of medicines being made from hormone-like substances obtained from your own gut bacteria, which then improve your metabolism. This was once a utopia, but before long it may be the basis for new medical treatments and the discovery of new hormones. While I don't believe improving our gut bacteria composition and diversity will resolve all of the world's diseases, I do expect it will give us better control of our hormonal balance.

A new generation of researchers will be able to rein in the power of hormones in our daily lives via interventions to the gut bacteria. As a result, an improved thyroid function could help reduce the severity of an autoimmune disease, for example, or an increased appetite could help patients undergoing cancer treatment. And there are many other conditions in which hormones are important for our physical and mental well-being and for which gut bacteria may be able to have a beneficial role. This is a fantastic prospect – thanks to Ge Hong and Dioscorides, who shared their insights more than two thousand years ago.

# 7

# Hormones Make or Break
# the Man and Woman

*Adulthood*

An American study in 2009 found that between 5 and 10 per cent of the adult population will be affected by an endocrine disease at some point.[1] These are mainly the usual suspects: diabetes and thyroid disorders, such as hypothyroidism. However, all endocrine disorders have a big impact on the disease burden and on the chance of survival of patients. If the endocrine glands no longer work effectively, you might think we could fix this by substituting the missing hormones with pills or injections. This is something we are able to do as doctors, but it doesn't magic the problem away. Medication is unable to simulate the natural regulation and production of hormones. It is the subtle interplay between body and endocrine system that is responsible for our well-being. Or, as Hilary Mantel put it in the Foreword to this book: if your hormonal balance changes, your mind changes too.[2]

In this chapter, we will take a closer look at the most common hormone treatments – starting with the contraceptive pill – and at endocrine disorders in adults.

## The birth of the contraceptive pill

During my time at the University of California in San Diego between 2007 and 2008, I enjoyed attending the weekly academic lunchtime seminars in which famous alumni like the businessman Craig Venter and Nobel Prize winner Paul Crutzen would tell their life stories, in shorts and flip-flops, to an interested and heterogenous audience in a well-filled auditorium. After the seminar, we were invited to have a chat with these luminaries over a cup of coffee.

It was at one of these events that I heard about Carl Djerassi, a well-known American scientist and writer who was involved in the development of the contraceptive pill in the 1950s. In his wonderful autobiography, *This Man's Pill*,[3] he evocatively describes how the discovery of the production of synthetic female hormone in the lab unfolded before his eyes. Yet he wonders, and rightly so, why a pill for men has not been developed. And why was it that in some countries, such as Japan, the pill wasn't available from doctors until the end of the 1990s?

However, Djerassi's main conclusion was that there wouldn't have been a sexual revolution without the contraceptive pill. Studies from the 1960s showed that frequent use of the hormones oestrogen and progestogen made a woman less fertile. This discovery came at a remarkably opportune moment: on the one hand, certain groups were warning of overpopulation in wealthy western Europe; on the other hand, feminists were keen to see women gain more control over the timing of their reproduction.

The modern contraceptive pill contains either just

progesterone, or both progesterone and oestrogen. These two hormones inhibit ovulation (see Chapter 1), which prevents fertilisation by a sperm cell. This is the best-known effect of 'the pill', but it can also be used for menstrual complaints such as heavy bleeding and for pre-menstrual syndrome (PMS). It is also used for patients with endometriosis, an often-undiagnosed condition in which endometrial tissue spreads through the ovaries and abdominal cavity. Endometriosis is associated with severe pain, and although treatment with the contraceptive pill reduces the symptoms, it doesn't address the root of the problem.

In 1995, Saskia Middeldorp, a professor of internal medicine in Nijmegen, Gelderland, whose field of research is thrombosis, raised the alarm when it emerged that the use of a certain pill led to an increased risk of thrombosis (clots in the blood vessels that can prove fatal). The consequence was a drastic decrease in the prescription of pills with high levels of oestrogen.[4] At the same time, people became more aware of other side effects of hormonal medications. Weight gain (due to additional oestrogen) and decreased libido are some of the most common complaints associated with taking the pill. It has been suspected for a long time that the pill reduces libido. This is probably because a lengthy period of hormonal 'supplementation' suppresses the production of your own sex hormones more and more, resulting in consistently high levels of progesterone and oestrogen, and fewer androgens, relatively speaking. This can have a significant impact on your body, in both positive and negative terms. Through the widespread, global use of the pill, these effects are becoming increasingly evident.[5]

A contraceptive pill containing progesterone could also lead to fatigue and mood changes. This can be a great burden for some women and reason enough to stop taking it. Some people are more susceptible to the negative effects of progesterone than others.[6] In a recent large-scale Danish study, the connection between depressive feelings and the use of female hormones was examined more extensively. Almost half a million women who used hormonal contraceptives were followed over a period of eight years. The researchers looked specifically at the risk of (attempted) suicide and compared the participants with a control group of women who had never used hormones.[7] The risk of attempted suicide proved significantly higher among users of the pill than the control group, and the effect was even more apparent in users of contraceptive pills containing progesterone. It's therefore clear that some women are especially susceptible to this hormone. Doctors are strongly advised to take risk factors into account when prescribing certain contraceptive pills.

Prolonged fatigue is one of the most common side effects of the contraceptive pill. This is related to a shortage of testosterone, which makes women feel less energetic.[8] The small amount of testosterone produced by the ovaries also decreases, because the hormones in the pill suppress the stimulation of this organ. A reduction of testosterone is sometimes actually the desired effect, for example if acne is the reason for taking the pill. And when you stop taking the pill, your own production of testosterone doesn't suddenly return to normal, which is why you can still feel tired months later.[9] Fortunately, if the pill doesn't work for you there are also other types of hormonal contraceptive, such as the hormonal shot or the coil, which are also effective at preventing a pregnancy but have far fewer side effects.

There is one unexpected and beneficial side effect of the pill, however. Women are known for having good memories; they remember details much better than men.[10] Research shows that this is influenced by the use of the contraceptive pill. In an experiment, women who did and didn't take the pill were shown films and then, a week later, asked what they could remember.

The women with a natural cycle remembered the emotional components much better, whereas those who were on the pill were able to summarise the story better, as men usually do.[11] From this, we can deduce that a natural hormonal balance helps you remember emotional details, but that the contraceptive pill focuses your attention more on the core of the matter. The ability to remember details isn't something to be proud of; it's all down to your hormones. Now we just need to remember this detail ourselves.

## If your immune system is compromised

I remember my first year of medical studies in Utrecht, in the mid-1990s. Standing in the dissecting room, with the penetrating odour of formalin in my nose (I could still smell it that night), I held them in my hand: a thyroid gland and two adrenal glands. They might be small, delicate organs, but they are incredibly important. Aristotle stated that the thyroid enables our soul to work better.[12] In adulthood (from the age of twenty to fifty), it is often the thyroid and the adrenal glands that cause most complaints. The hormones they produce have a direct effect on the brain, energy levels, metabolism and the immune system – all of the tissues and cells that protect your body against intruders such as bacteria and viruses. And if your immune system isn't functioning properly, it can't do what it is meant to do: keep pathogens out.

That doesn't go unnoticed: think, for example, of winter viruses or chronic problems such as high blood pressure. We have some understanding of flu and we recently also become acquainted with COVID-19. What's less well known is the role that hormones play in our defence against these viruses. Chronically elevated levels of cortisol, for example, make us more susceptible to viral infections, and also more infectious to other people.[13] Day after day, various hormonal substances work together to keep our blood pressure under control and to prevent us from fainting. These hormones are vitally important behind the scenes.

Often, we only realise that something is wrong when the endocrine system becomes unbalanced. Gradually, symptoms start to develop that can lead to illness. Complaints vary from physical (weight gain) to mental (depression) and from mild (muscular pain) to serious (death). Hormonal disorders in adulthood are sometimes caused by the deterioration of a hormone-producing gland, but they're more likely to be caused by a process brought on by an autoimmune disease. This is when your immune system attacks the somatic cells in your hormone-producing glands and damages them. If, for example, you have an underactive thyroid gland (hypothyroidism), you produce antibodies that break down your thyroid gland and lead to scarring. As a result, your thyroid gland slows down and you often need treatment with synthetically made thyroid hormone in the form of pills.[14] Doctors still don't know exactly how to detect a malfunctioning hormone gland at an early stage, and by the time the disease manifests itself, it is often already too late. That's why some patients need medical treatment for their entire lives. In the next sections, I will explain how exactly that works, starting with the thyroid gland.

## Underactive or overactive thyroid

The thyroid is located just in front of the larynx and produces the hormone thyroxin (T4), which is involved in a whole host of important metabolic processes in the body. T4 regulates body temperature and metabolism (how the body obtains energy

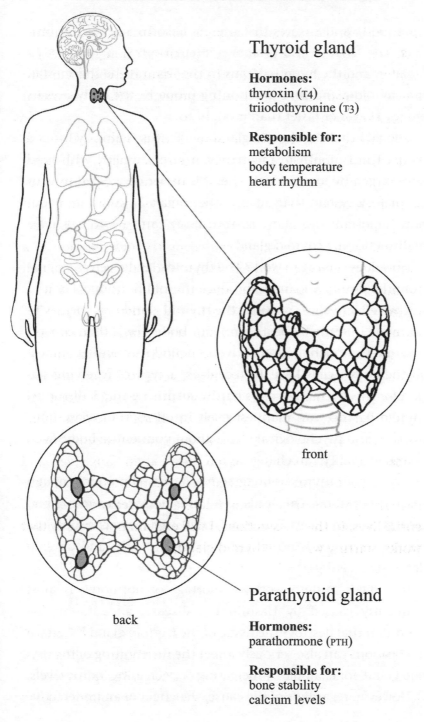

## Thyroid gland

**Hormones:**
thyroxin (T4)
triiodothyronine (T3)

**Responsible for:**
metabolism
body temperature
heart rhythm

front

back

## Parathyroid gland

**Hormones:**
parathormone (PTH)

**Responsible for:**
bone stability
calcium levels

from food), and ensures that the gut absorbs and burns nutrients. The thyroid also promotes circulation; it is your body's radiator, and the hypothalamus in the brain is the thermostat. If a thyroid gland isn't functioning properly, the body uses its energy slower or faster than it ought to.

The fact that the thyroid gland of a foetus is already formed in the third month of pregnancy, and is supplied with food and oxygen by four arteries – i.e. it is better connected to your circulatory system than many other organs – says a lot about how important this gland is. Your body can't afford to have a malfunctioning thyroid gland.

How does this organ work? The thyroid gland receives a signal from the pituitary gland to produce thyroid hormone. For it to work as effectively as possible, the thyroid gland first releases T4 hormone into the bloodstream. Your body's cells then convert this into the much more effective T3 (triiodothyronine). Almost all the body's cells have T3 receptors, a type of receiving station for this hormone, so it's hardly surprising that a disrupted thyroid balance can manifest itself in all sorts of ways, both physical and psychological, throughout your entire body. Even your personality can change as a result.

If your thyroid is underactive, it doesn't produce enough thyroid hormone. This leads to a lower body temperature and cold hands and feet. You may also suffer from constipation, because your gut is no longer working properly, and develop depressive feelings.[15]

In today's western world, a shortage of hormones is most frequently caused by Hashimoto's disease, an autoimmune condition that destroys the tissue of the thyroid gland.[16] Certain medications can also seriously affect the functioning of the thyroid gland, for example by increasing or decreasing iodine levels.

However, regardless of the cause, the effect of an underactive thyroid is always the same: patients suffer from weight gain, a lower heart rate, dry skin, hair loss and concentration problems. Strangely enough, this affects some people greatly and others barely at all. I once saw a patient in my clinic whose thyroid barely produced any hormone, but who had run a half marathon with ease, aside from some muscle pain. At the same time, another patient with a slight anomaly of the thyroid gland had so many complaints that he was signed off work sick. Doctors also observe that the outcome of treatment can vary dramatically, depending on the patient.

On the other hand, a thyroid gland can also be overactive (hyperthyroidism), which can result in weight loss and hyperactivity and is sometimes associated with psychiatric complaints such as mania. An overactive thyroid is often enlarged and sometimes the eye muscles are swollen, which leads to bulging eyes. In most cases, the immune system is partially behind any change to the way the thyroid gland normally works – for example with Graves' disease, also called Basedow's disease. Art connoisseurs may be familiar with the characteristic neck swelling (goitre) in Mantegna's *Madonna with Sleeping Child* or Caravaggio's *Madonna of the Rosary*.[17] This can be caused by either an underactive or overactive thyroid. It is believed that the Greek philosopher Socrates also suffered from this.[18]

The American president George Bush Sr and his wife Barbara both showed symptoms of having an overactive thyroid. When their dog developed similar complaints, the CIA launched an investigation into the iodine level in the family's immediate surroundings. Unfortunately the United States Secret Service didn't share the results, but it's rumoured that Bush's illness affected his mood to such an extent that it impacted the decisions he made as president.[19] He ordered the invasion of Iraq in 1991 even though his advisors had urged him not to, for example, and his relatives found his behaviour peculiar. After aggressive medical treatment, not only was his thyroid function exhausted, but also his desire for war. The American troops were withdrawn ahead of time and that's probably why the severely fatigued president was not re-elected.

# A brief history

Leonardo da Vinci was the first to depict the thyroid gland, around the year 1500.[20] In 1543, the Flemish doctor Andreas Vesalius included the thyroid gland in his *De humani corporis fabrica libri septem*, a set of seven books about the structure of the human body. A century later, the English anatomist Thomas Wharton, a fellow at the Royal London College of Physicians, wrote about the importance of this gland for our temperature and mood in his anatomy book *Adenographia*, published in 1656.[21] Around fourteen hundred years earlier, the thyroid was already considered an important organ, although people were not aware of its function. In the second century after Christ, the Greek-Roman doctor Claudius Galen, who dominated medical science for centuries with his theories about the human body, was the first to call the gland the *thyroides*, after the Greek word for 'shield'. Galen believed that due to its strategic position in the neck, the quadrilateral cartilage constituted a connection between heart and soul, and that it could protect the physical from the mental (and vice versa), like a type of border control.

Although the actual function of the thyroid gland was only discovered relatively recently through medical research, people who suffered from thyroid problems can be seen in ancient illustrations. The Egyptian pharaoh Tutankhamun, who lived in the fourteenth century BC, appeared to have a swelling on his neck, as did the Egyptian Queen Cleopatra (69–31 BC). The effects of anomalies of the thyroid gland fascinated physicians, philosophers and artists all over the world, from Ancient Greece to India and from China to Egypt. In the second century BC, the Chinese effectively treated thyroid diseases with sponge-like animals, which we now know contain high levels of iodine.[22] As we discovered in the previous chapter, Dioscorides also experimented with faecal transplantations in an attempt to improve thyroid function.

To discover the function of an organ, doctors try to identify its tissue type. The cells designated for the thyroid are formed at an early stage in the development of a foetus from the so-called branchial apparatus; in fish and amphibians, this is the place responsible for the development of the gills. It was only in the nineteenth and twentieth centuries that we gained greater insight into the thyroid gland. In 1895, the German researcher Eugen Baumann carried out an experiment in which he boiled the thyroid tissue of a good thousand sheep and used this preparation to successfully treat people with thyroid abnormalities. In order to better understand the thyroid, he observed the behaviour of dogs and monkeys whose thyroid glands he had surgically removed.[23] In 1852, the French doctor Adolphe Chatin was the first to suggest a link between goitre and iodine deficiency. He transported salt from regions with few thyroid patients to regions where thyroid disease was especially prevalent.[24] He did this because a colleague of his had just discovered that sea salt contained a purple substance called iodine, named after the Greek word for the colour purple: *ioeides*. And guess what? Salt solved most of the problems of the thyroid patients. However, goitre as a result of an iodine deficiency remained a common problem in remote areas until well into the nineteenth century. In the Netherlands, it took a good century before iodized salt found its way to the table and before iodine was routinely added to bread dough.[25]

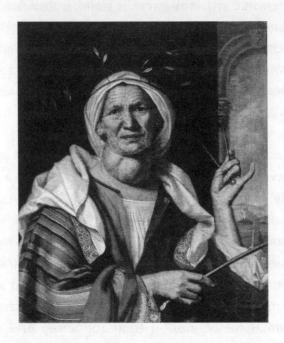

Painting by Pietro Bellotti (1627–1700) depicting a dowser
with an enlarged thyroid gland (goitre)

The first treatment using thyroid hormone came to the market in 1949. The Dutch company Organon was one of several companies that began manufacturing medications containing thyroid hormone obtained from the waste material of slaughtered animals. One of these substances (thyreoidum) is still available on the market and, due to the predominantly natural source of the hormone, is popular among practitioners of alternative medicine. The varying composition of these pills can be problematic for the body, but that's fortunately not the case with synthetically produced thyroid tablets. Over-the-counter diet pills and products made from slaughterhouse waste are known to pose a risk to the thyroid gland because they respond to characteristics of thyroid hormone that cause your metabolism and fat-burning to go into overdrive.[26] Likewise, animal products are associated with *thyrotoxicosis factitia*, a disorder whereby you are 'poisoned' by an overdose of thyroid hormone in your bloodstream. This is why the contamination of beef mince with animal thyroid hormone led to outbreaks of thyroid disease, also known as 'hamburger thyrotoxicosis', in the 1980s.[27]

## Stress and thyroid problems

In the case of George Bush Sr, the office of president and the associated long-term stress potentially led to him developing Graves' disease, causing his thyroid to go wild and his mental health to deteriorate. A hormonal disorder can influence our mood, but serious, long-term psychological stress can also impact our hormonal balance and even result in disease.[28]

In war zones, for example, there is a clear link between stress and thyroid problems. World wars and civil wars are characterised by periods in which large groups of people are exposed to extreme stress for a long time. After the First World War, doctors and researchers saw a sudden increase in thyroid problems among former soldiers and citizens from war zones.[29] After the Second World War, a new peak in cases of thyroid disease was observed. Previously, there had only been a few thyroid problems in Germany's Black Forest region, but after the war doctors diagnosed a larger number of people with overactive thyroids.[30] The same phenomenon occurred in the Balkans around the time of the Yugoslav Wars in the 1990s.[31]

The link between stress and the thyroid was first made almost two hundred years before those wars. In an article published in 1825, the British doctor Caleb Hillier Parry described a

21-year-old patient who had developed an overactive thyroid a number of weeks after she had fallen out of a wheelchair and suffered from a major shock.[32] In 1840, the German doctor Carl von Basedow reported the case of a man with hyperthyroidism after a period of stress resulting from business conflicts.[33] The Irish doctor Robert James Graves had discovered the same autoimmune condition somewhat earlier: both are considered to have discovered what is now known as Graves' disease, or Basedow disease.

Scientific journals frequently report similar cases. One of the most fascinating of these was described in 2009 in an offshoot of *Nature*. Italian researchers presented the case of an eighteen-year-old woman who had developed an overactive thyroid as a result of stressful life events. They showed how sedative medication (benzodiazepines) had been able to reduce the severity of her condition.[34] This is especially interesting because we generally use medication to treat the thyroid, whereas this shows that treating physical stress with tranquilisers can also indirectly have a beneficial effect on the thyroid function itself.

Another example of the influence of stress on the thyroid often reveals itself after giving birth – a stressful event for the body – as inflammation of the thyroid gland known as postpartum thyroiditis. In this condition, the thyroid first produces an excessive amount of T4 thyroid hormone, which makes the patient feel agitated, and then it produces too little, which causes her to feel tired and lethargic. Given that most women feel tired after giving birth, coupled with the ensuing sleepless nights, this condition is often overlooked by doctors. Fortunately, the thyroid function usually recovers within a year and this condition appears to be a manifestation of the physical stress that a pregnancy entails.[35]

If your immune system attacks your body's own cells, this is referred to as an autoimmune condition. As mentioned earlier, most endocrine conditions in adults are caused by this autoimmune process. Graves' disease is not unique in this respect.[36] Other glands can be affected in a similar manner, like the pancreas (type 1 diabetes), adrenal glands (Addison's disease), ovaries (POI or premature menopause) and sometimes even several organs at the same time. In 1901, before these endocrine diseases were officially discovered, the German Nobel Prize winner and immunologist Paul Ehrlich described them as 'horror autotoxicus', referring to the horror of self-poisoning, which says a lot about the severity of the symptoms.[37] Various treatments are available to manage the symptoms, but unfortunately autoimmune conditions are incurable. Researchers are busy searching for the causes of these diseases and ways to influence their progression.

Strikingly, autoimmune conditions are almost nine times more common in women than men. Research shows that female sex hormones, oestrogens, stimulate certain immune cells in the body, which causes the endocrine glands to wear out, whereas testosterone has a curbing effect.[38] After the menopause, women are less likely to develop autoimmune conditions; they have lower oestrogen levels because this hormone is no longer produced during the menopause. That's why their immune system behaves more like a male immune system. This proves, yet again, that hormones influence the work of the immune system.[39]

In recent decades, the number of people with an autoimmune condition has almost doubled globally, while male and female hormone levels have remained relatively stable. It therefore seems likely that external influences cause or exacerbate these diseases, including medication or changes to our (western) diet, which is often ultra-processed and packed full of preservatives.[40]

Excessive hygiene measures can also cause problems; your immune system becomes less 'experienced' as a result.

And then there are the key players mentioned in the previous chapter that try to curb the external influences on your immune system: gut bacteria. They work closely together with your immune cells, the majority of which are located in your gut, in the small intestine. Proper training is required for the development of an experienced immune system that responds to intruders but leaves its own cells alone. Some gut bacteria are especially important for specific parts of this immune cell training.[41] An effective composition of the intestinal flora may protect you against immune disorders – Dioscorides was on the right track with his dog poo treatment for thyroid complaints two thousand years ago.

Researching the interplay between gut bacteria and the production of hormones appears to be increasingly necessary in identifying both the cause and the development of endocrine disorders. Hopefully, a greater understanding of this in the near future will lead to new treatment methods.

## Adrenal glands

The adrenal glands are located just above the kidneys. They are as small as a segment of orange – and weigh just eight grams in total – but produce five different hormones: aldosterone, adrenaline, cortisol, testosterone and noradrenaline. The main function of these hormones is to help us respond effectively to stress: they raise our blood pressure, make us more alert and give us more energy. In periods of rest, such as after a workout or a busy day, the adrenal glands produce hormones that contribute to physical recovery, such as cortisol. In short, an adult needs effective adrenal glands in order to stay healthy.

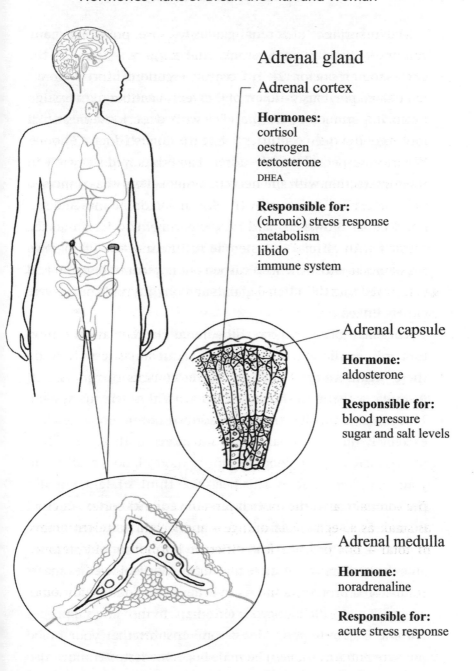

**Adrenal gland**

Adrenal cortex

**Hormones:**
cortisol
oestrogen
testosterone
DHEA

**Responsible for:**
(chronic) stress response
metabolism
libido
immune system

Adrenal capsule

**Hormone:**
aldosterone

**Responsible for:**
blood pressure
sugar and salt levels

Adrenal medulla

**Hormone:**
noradrenaline

**Responsible for:**
acute stress response

The importance of adrenal glands was overlooked for many centuries. Pioneers in anatomy and surgery – such as the Greek-Roman doctor Galen from the second century, whom I mentioned previously – knew of their existence but didn't assign much importance to the gland described as 'loose flesh'.[42] It took a good sixteen centuries before the English doctor Thomas Wharton suspected that the adrenal glands played a key role in their interaction with the nervous system. This was confirmed in the nineteenth century by the British doctor Thomas Addison and Charles Brown-Séquard (yes, the same man who injected himself with animal testosterone to increase his libido), two big names in medicine who carried out important research and discovered that the adrenal glands and physical well-being were closely linked.

The small but very powerful adrenal glands play an important role in the event of physical or mental stress. How do these organs work? Their inner layer consists of the adrenal medulla, a tissue in direct contact with the nervous system. This explains why it can produce adrenaline and noradrenaline extremely quickly in dangerous situations. Both of these hormones increase your blood pressure so more blood is available to your brain and muscles. This helps you think straight, but also perform better. In the outer layer – the adrenal cortex – steroid hormones such as cortisol, aldosterone and testosterone are produced. Cortisol, also known as the 'stress hormone', is probably the best known of these hormones. Cortisol releases sugars from stored proteins and fats in order to generate (additional) energy. It also influences your circadian rhythm and suppresses chronic inflammation. Aldosterone ensures that your blood pressure remains stable. The male hormone testosterone is also produced here. All of these hormones are generated from cholesterol (from food and by the liver) and can therefore be easily transported through the body. Cholesterol is hydrophobic, but it's also the basis of the cell membranes in our body, which is why the hormones can easily reach the inside of each cell to do their work. If cholesterol calcifies the artery wall then this can cause cardiovascular diseases, as it slowly blocks blood flow in the arteries.

The hormones noradrenaline and adrenaline work differently; they come from the core of your adrenal gland, which is directly linked to your central nervous system. When these hormones are produced, your body acts reflexively, before you can even think about it. This is what happens when, for example, you touch a hot pan. Within a few seconds of the first signs of stress, the quantity of adrenaline and noradrenaline in your blood increases. This improves your ability to react and you get a boost of energy. It is hardly surprising that adrenaline was found to be a mood enhancer.

The British politician Anthony Eden was completely crazy about adrenaline, in the 1950s. Before he became prime minister, he had taken the stimulant Benzedrine, a type of amphetamine that is very similar to adrenaline, in connection with an operation. Perhaps his new job was too much for him to handle, because he continued taking the performance-enhancing amphetamine pills in secret.[43] These 'bennies' were very popular at that time. In the case of Eden, who was usually so mindful, the use of these pills led to recklessness and excessive self-confidence. The price for that would be paid during the Suez crisis, the conflict around ownership and access to the Suez Canal, with Egypt on one side and Israel, France and the United Kingdom on the other. Eden's attitude towards the Egyptian president Nasser surprised friend and foe alike when, in 1956, the British politician decided – without the support of the US as its biggest ally – to invade the Suez Canal. According to his biography, this decision could be attributed to the effect of the substance on his hormones. The Suez crisis accelerated Britain's decline as a major power, and the disillusioned Eden was forced to resign.

The importance of proper adrenal function is still under-estimated today. This was apparent during the coronavirus pandemic, when doctors prescribed the synthetic (adrenal) stress hormone dexamethasone in an attempt to increase survival rates for COVID-19 patients.[44]

If your adrenal glands aren't functioning properly, they are either overactive or underactive and are producing too many or too few hormones. Underactive adrenal glands are seen in the event of chronic stress. If they have to work extremely hard over a long period of time, they wear out and lose the ability to coordinate with the rest of the body. You could compare this to an overstretched elastic band, which no longer returns to its original shape. As a result, your adrenal glands produce insuffi-cient hormones and this is very noticeable: you wake up feeling tired, have a poor memory, have a high blood sugar level, feel stressed and are oversensitive.[45] These symptoms are all also characteristics of burnout. Cortisol does appear to play a role in burnout, although there's not yet an effective test to show the extent to which the adrenal gland has been thrown off kilter when these symptoms are present. Hopefully further research will help us better understand this connection in future.

If you have the rare autoimmune condition Addison's dis-ease, on the other hand, your adrenal glands produce too few hormones because of an infection. Your immune system then turns against your adrenal glands (as is the case with an under-active thyroid); the organs become damaged and produce less cortisol and aldosterone. As a result, you feel exhausted, down, crave salty foods, and your skin and mucous membranes turn darker, as if you have spent a long time in the sun. You also lose a significant amount of weight. If this happens, you can use exogenous cortisol, such as dexamethasone or hydrocortisone, to compensate for the deficit. This can be administered as tablets or injections. Today, this type of treatment is tailored precisely to the individual body's requirements.

This hasn't always been the case. The American president John F. Kennedy, like his sister Eunice, suffered from Addison's disease. Doctors established he had the rare disease when he was thirty years old, so a long time before his presidency. At that time, hormone therapy was still in its infancy, and the treatment he received led to serious fluctuations in the cortisol levels in his blood. Before important events, Kennedy's personal physician Max Jacobson, whose nickname 'Dr Feelgood' says it all, really, would boost these levels by means of corticosteroid injections (combined with a considerable amount of testosterone). But this tinkering with synthetic hormones went awry in the run-up to the Cuba crisis in 1961. When the Soviet leader Nikita Khrushchev turned up very late to a political meeting with the American president, he was met by an overtired Kennedy who simply sat there like a wet rag, barely able to formulate sentences. The unfortunate timing meant it was too long since the president had received his cortisol shot.[46] A president who was secretly being injected with mind-altering drugs (including testosterone and cortisol) at the most dangerous time in the Cold War: historians believe it's possible that the failed diplomatic negotiations raised tensions, resulting in the nuclear missiles aimed at Cuba being called off at the very last minute and a nuclear war only narrowly being averted.

The pigment formation was clearly visible in JFK, who often sported a nice tan. Charisma always works well during a presidential election and the fact that presidential candidate Richard

Nixon literally paled beside Kennedy during the television debate in 1960 likely contributed to Kennedy's victory.[47]

On top of the signs of exhaustion and his 'White House tan', JFK also had various physical complaints due to an imbalance between his thyroid hormones and sex hormones. During his presidency, his health further deteriorated, although this was not disclosed to the public until long after his death. Whether or not Dr Feelgood's daily shots influenced his notorious womanising behaviour – he had several affairs during his marriage – remains unclear, but it's certainly not inconceivable.[48]

Adrenal glands can also work too *hard*. This could be a temporary consequence of stress, in which case it's not harmful. But if your adrenal glands produce too many hormones (in surges), your body ends up in trouble and could develop an adrenal gland tumour, for example. Lesser-known consequences of the adrenal glands being in overdrive include phaeochromocytoma – when too much adrenaline causes palpitations, sweating and headaches – and Conn's syndrome, when too much aldosterone leads to raised blood pressure. The most recognisable risk is the adrenal gland tumour that results in an excess of cortisol: Cushing's syndrome, named after the American neurosurgeon Harvey Cushing. As cortisol influences other (endocrine) processes in your body, you can end up with a whole host of symptoms if you have too much of this hormone in your bloodstream: an increase in fat mass, the absence of menstruation (in women), reduced libido (in men), raised blood pressure, chronic fatigue and muscle weakness.

A 23-year-old patient called Minnie, whom Cushing examined in 1910, triggered his interest in the syndrome; she exhibited all of the above-mentioned symptoms of excessive exposure to cortisol.[49] Minnie's complaints inspired Cushing to conduct a lengthy investigation into the cause of chronically elevated cortisol levels in the bloodstream, which remains puzzling today. One thing we do know is that Cushing's syndrome can be fatal if left untreated. Minnie lived for a good forty years after her diagnosis. Doctors and patients should be very grateful to Cushing for his research.

## Yoga and breathing to alleviate stress

Let's return to stress. Our bodies are designed to switch 'on' in the event of stress. In the past, when we were regularly at risk of great danger, a quick reaction could literally save our lives. But a great deal has changed since then. We are now exposed to completely different stressors and the trick is to retain the positive aspects of stress while leaving the negative ones behind. Stress does have its advantages, as Sonia Lupien writes in her book *Well Stressed*.[50] Stress from time pressure or great responsibility can lead to improved performance, as long as this stress isn't perceived as chronic. Otherwise, accumulated stress tries to find another way out, and you soon find yourself having to deal with the hormonal consequences.

---

### The discovery of a miracle cure

In the twentieth century, discoveries were made for which Nobel Prizes were awarded. But only one of these discoveries involved a 'miracle' cure. Exceptionally, the researchers were awarded this international accolade within two years of the first use of this substance. As with many great discoveries, coincidence played a key role.[51]

---

In the spring of 1929, the American rheumatologist Philip Hench noticed that the symptoms of a patient who suffered from a serious form of rheumatoid arthritis disappeared after an episode of jaundice (a liver condition). As there was no treatment for rheumatoid arthritis at that time, this aroused his interest. In the following years, Hench observed the same phenomenon in other patients with rheumatoid arthritis, but attempts to treat it with liver-like tissue came to nothing.

In the meantime, it had emerged that complaints associated with rheumatoid arthritis sometimes decreased after a pregnancy or surgical intervention. In both cases, the level of stress hormone in the bloodstream increased, and this insight led Hench to see if it was due to a mystery substance, and find out what it was. The fatigue experienced by patients with rheumatoid arthritis reminded him of the lethargy experienced by patients with the adrenal gland condition Addison's disease. He decided to contact the biochemist Edward Kendall, who had managed to successfully isolate thyroid hormone and was now carrying out research into the function of the adrenal gland. The pair of scientists received help from an unexpected source.

In 1941, the US was on the cusp of entering the Second World War. It was rumoured that the Nazis were collecting animal adrenal tissue in order to lift the spirits of their soldiers and increase their resistance to stress. It turned out that they were using Benzedrine, the same pill that would cost Anthony Eden his presidency twenty years later.[52] Studies had shown that stress proved fatal for animals without adrenal glands. The researchers therefore suspected that the hormones produced by these glands offered protection against stress.

The US decided to invest millions of dollars in the research and production of active stress substances. Many years later, Hench and Kendall successfully isolated a corticosteroid that is produced in the adrenal cortex and has a powerful anti-inflammatory effect. It is now known as prednisone.

The success of the present-day treatment with prednisone, the most effective medication for rheumatoid arthritis, is primarily thanks to an assertive patient, Mrs Gardner. She had suffered from serious rheumatoid arthritis for many years and used a wheelchair. In 1948, she stayed on Philip Hench's ward for a while and refused to leave the hospital until he had cured her. She insisted that she be used as a guinea pig for treatment with the synthetically produced stress hormone cortisone (referred to as 'compound E' at that time). She already felt better by the third day and after a week, all of her symptoms had disappeared.[53] Other patients were given the same substance and it proved effective for all of them. It made global headlines and corticosteroids are still used for various diseases to this day, despite the many side effects.

Mrs Gardner died six years after her 'miracle' cure. The excessive dosage of cortisone gave her serious physical and psychological symptoms resembling Cushing's syndrome.

Up to a quarter of the world's population regularly suffers from anxiety and feelings of depression.[54] It's hardly surprising that stress also has a huge psychological impact if you consider how well attuned your body is to react to danger. Receptors for stress hormones are present throughout your body, including in your brain, which is why long-term stress also affects your memory, attention span and emotions. The popularity of age-old methods to reduce stress, such as acupuncture and yoga, isn't entirely coincidental.[55]

But how effective are these 'alternative' therapies? Researchers found that cortisol levels improved in people who regularly performed breathing exercises or practised yoga.[56,57] As cortisol increases blood sugar levels – the body needs more energy to avoid danger – diabetes patients also appear to benefit from the ancient Indian form of movement. A large-scale study revealed that daily yoga exercises helped improve blood sugar levels, resulting in lower levels in the morning and more stable levels after meals.[58] But the influence of yoga on the body is not limited to the hormone cortisol. Cortisol and sugar levels are, for their part, involved in the development of polycystic ovarian syndrome, mentioned in Chapter 1, which is a common cause of infertility in (often overweight) young women, who have ovulation problems. It emerged that yoga stimulated the production of sex hormones in these women, making them menstruate more frequently (and probably also increasing fertility).

Yoga has also been shown to influence growth hormones in older age as well as thyroid levels in women who produce too little thyroid hormone.[59] Due to these physical *and* mental benefits, yoga is cautiously suggested as a type of 'hormone therapy'.[60] However, further research is needed to determine whether it can actually be utilised for chronic endocrine disorders, and if so, how that would work.

## Hormones are cash: anabolic steroids

At the start of the twentieth century, it became clear that hormonal substances have a major influence on our physical attributes. An international race ensued between pharmaceutical companies and researchers to become the first to isolate and industrially manufacture an active hormone. The Amsterdam-based research team at Organon, led by the pharmacologist Ernst Laquer, founder of endocrinology in the Netherlands, the endocrinologist Marius Tausk and the chemist Lize Dingemanse, discovered female oestrogens a fraction too late; the US future Nobel Prize winner Edward Doisy just beat them to it when he first isolated the hormones in 1929, and in 1938 created an oestrogen treatment (Femarin). In the case of testosterone, however, Laquer's team made a world premiere in 1935.[61] This was a nice twist of fate for the professor, who was known as a womaniser (and perhaps enjoyed sampling his homemade male hormone from time to time).[62]

The entrepreneurial spirit of Saal van Zwanenberg, a butcher from Oss in the Dutch province of North Brabant, was at least equally important for this triumph. As he had been looking for a way to earn money from animal tissue remains, there was a constant supply of tissue for hormone research when the successful company Organon was founded in 1923. This enabled the Dutch work to progress much more rapidly. Later, Laquer's team managed to isolate the female hormone progesterone from this material, and Organon became known for the development of an early version of the contraceptive pill. Organon also succeeded in producing a synthetic variant of the thyroid hormone, which they called Thryax. But it was Organon's large-scale production of testosterone that made the headlines. Thanks to this discovery, the substance was being produced in laboratories by 1935. Strikingly, it wasn't the Jewish pharmacologist Laqueur, but the German chemist Adolf Butenandt who was awarded the Nobel Prize in 1939 for his work on sex hormones.[63]

In order to understand how this discovery was made, we need to return to 1896, when the Austrian physiologists Zoth and Pregl repeated Brown-Séquard's experiment on themselves, but with a better, higher-quality solution. Although they didn't yet know which substance in the animal testicles was responsible for it, they established that their injections had a beneficial long-term effect when combined with intensive exercise.[64] In an attempt to measure differences in the degree of fatigue before and after the injections, they used a mechanical instrument from Italy: Mosso's ergograph. This instrument records the number of times in a row you can lift a small weight with one finger. When it emerged that their performances improved, Zoth and Pregl suggested that sportspeople could benefit from this 'organotherapy', the first form of doping! Adolf Hitler (referred to as 'Patient A') also received injections from his personal doctor, Doctor Morell, which contained a concoction of bulls' hearts and livers, mixed with amphetamine, designed to boost his testosterone levels and give him more energy and courage.[65]

Half a century later, the Armenian chemist Charles Kochakian administered hormone injections to dogs. His research proved that testosterone sets anabolic, androgenic processes in motion: anabolic because the hormone stimulates muscle growth, and androgenic because the hormone remains inextricably linked with masculine features.[66] While doctors and scientists saw opportunities for patients with protein loss (caused by burns or muscular diseases, for example), the sporting world argued the opposite: giving testosterone to people without a deficit of it could considerably speed up muscle gain. In the 1954 world weightlifting championships in Austria, it was the Russians, a team of remarkably hairy giants, who took home all the prizes. After a couple of glasses of vodka with his Russian colleague, the American team doctor John Ziegler discovered the secret: testosterone. Injections of this male hormone had, in a very short space of time, led to unprecedented muscle mass gains in the competitors.[67] Ziegler saw the potential of such injections for weightlifters and took the idea back with him to the US, where pharmaceutical companies invested in the development of the ideal bodybuilding pill. If you physically exert yourself over a long period of time, your body automatically makes hormones like cortisol and testosterone, which help build muscle. The injections were a way to enhance these effects.

Ziegler achieved effective results with the first versions of his testosterone injections that he administered to himself and other bodybuilders, but he soon became aware of the drug's side effects.[68] His own team struggled with liver problems and not long afterwards it emerged that the Russian athletes had developed such large prostates that they were only able to urinate with the help of a catheter. The athletes also appeared to have become dependent on the substances. Against Ziegler's medical advice, they continued to increase the dosage. The doctor soon advised against the use of the drugs and, until his death – caused by heart problems that he attributed to earlier doping – he maintained that introducing the drugs in sport had been a dark page in his life's story: a page he would like to have ripped out entirely.

As it has since been shown that testosterone tends to promote muscle *growth* as opposed to muscle *strength*,[69] it is primarily popular among amateur bodybuilders, for whom muscular form is at least as important as muscular function. In order to get an idea of the influence of testosterone use in this group, you only have to look at the evolution of boys' toys. Whereas GI Joe was still a lightweight action figure in the 1960s, fifty years later he is virtually bursting out of his own biceps.[70]

This culturally determined ideal of the everyday Mr Universe has contributed to an estimated one in ten gymgoers suffering from 'bigorexia': a fixation on building muscle mass. Although 'stacking' (taking more than one supplement at once) has proved very effective, it is not without risk. A study from 2014 showed that athletes who used these types of methods were three to four times more likely to die prematurely, usually between the ages of thirty and fifty.[71] The heart in particular doesn't cope well with hormonal overkill. Heart attacks and heart failure were diagnosed as the cause of death up to fifteen times more often in this group than in non-athletes of the same age.[72]

The natural steroids your body makes during prolonged exercise can, in themselves, have negative consequences too. Athletes can, for example, suffer from hair loss even if they don't take steroids, as seen in some Dutch professional football players. The difference is that the misuse of freely available androgens in excessively high dosages over time disrupts your whole endocrine system. The consequences can be far-reaching, including infertility and the development of mammary glands in men. An excess of male hormone therefore causes you to become *less* manly! This is because your own body tries to convert that excess testosterone into female hormones: oestrogens. These hormone injections also inhibit the production of the body's own testosterone, causing the testicles to become smaller. This is usually a temporary effect, but it is sometimes permanent.

Anyone who thinks that testosterone is only important for reproduction is clearly mistaken. The use of anabolic steroids is no longer limited to top athletes. In the US, many high school students have discovered that alongside Ritalin, a 'breakfast of champions' (the popular term for the steroid methandrostenolone, or Dianabol, which Ziegler also gave his athletes) also helps increase their concentration levels. Despite numerous warnings from the scientific community, the global consumption of these anabolic steroids is continuing to increase.[73]

Attempts to ban anabolic steroids raised awareness of the use of these substances in the livestock farming sector, where they're used to help veal calves or pigs rapidly gain weight and are sometimes easier or cheaper to obtain than products for human use. This has not been without its consequences. Since 1988, the importation of American beef has been prohibited in the EU in connection with high levels of active steroid hormones and the associated risks to public health.[74] Blood analysis revealed that the hormone values of an eight-year-old increased by 10 per cent after eating just two hamburgers.

Of course, taking synthetic or animal testosterone influences the human psyche. When people take exogenous steroids like prednisone, they often feel like they're on top of the world. This euphoria can backfire, however, if you take these anabolic steroids over a longer period of time. Well-known side effects include negative feelings, mood swings, fits of rage and aggressive behaviour. In the 1980s, when anabolic steroids were very popular among body builders, the number of criminal offences committed by members of this group increased. In many cases, lawyers argued temporary insanity based on steroid use, a defence referred to as 'roid rage' (roid is slang for steroid). This approach led to a reduced sentence on more than one occasion.

The best-known case related to the use of steroids and aggression is that of Oscar Pistorius, the 'Blade Runner', who murdered his girlfriend in 2013. When the police searched his house, they found supplies of anabolic steroids; Pistorius admitted feeling agitated that evening. However, it wasn't possible to prove a direct causal link between the use of steroids and such levels of aggression, so the theory could not be substantiated, even when the high levels of testosterone in the South African's blood were taken into consideration. Pistorius was found guilty and – partly due to contradictory statements about the reason for his possession of doping substances – received not a reduction, but a doubling of his sentence.

# The Power of Hormones

It's clear that you can't replace or even simulate the body's own functions by administering hormones. Playing around with hormone preparations yourself can also be dangerous, especially without medical supervision. It's therefore the doctor's job to not only find better treatment options, but also to detect endocrine disorders well before they manifest themselves in adulthood.

# 8

# The Change

*For Women* and *Men*

*Menopause The Musical* has been running in Las Vegas for fifteen years with great success. The show follows four women and contains virtually all the stereotypes associated with the menopause: they sing about chocolate, memory loss, night sweats, hot flushes and, of course, changes in their sex life. In the Netherlands, Yvonne van den Hurk's play about the menopause, *Hormonologen*, has also been a sell-out success.

Around 1.8 million Dutch women between the ages of forty and sixty are going through the menopause transition. In the UK that number is as high as 13 million. And men also experience all kinds of changes to their bodies at around the age of fifty. Here too, hormones play a key role. In this chapter I will explain a bit more about the menopause and the andropause. What exactly happens to your sex hormones during this phase and how do these changes make themselves known? How do we view the change: what did people make of it in the past and how is it perceived in other cultures? What can you do to get through this period the best way possible? Which hormone treatments are available for the symptoms?

Because the effects of the change are, in general, more significant for women than men, I will start with the menopause.

## Menopause: the last egg

Contrary to men, women don't produce new reproductive cells throughout their lives. This means they have to make do with a total supply of around 5 million egg cells; this figure starts decreasing from the moment of conception. By birth, they are left with 1.2 million, and by the start of puberty, 'only' three hundred thousand remain.[1] The older you become, the faster the number and quality of these cells declines. From the age of forty, your eggs drop in number until you run out completely around ten years later. This phase, the menopause, commonly starts around the age of fifty and lasts between one and two years. During this period, the cycle becomes increasingly irregular and the gaps between periods increase, before finally stopping altogether. The menopause is literally your very last menstruation; after that, the egg cells (follicles) have all been used up. You can only determine exactly when your menstrual cycle stopped a year later. The perimenopause (also referred to as the menopause transition) is the transitional time around menopause.

In the run-up to the last menstruation, various signs of hormonal fluctuations can often already be found in the blood. The ovaries age and the pituitary gland responds to this by producing more LH and FSH, causing oestrogen levels to go from a regular peak and trough to chaotically spiking and plummeting. These erratic spikes and falls ultimately end with oestrogens disappearing from the body, causing the range of hormones to change drastically; because there are no longer any follicles and therefore no egg cells either, the oestrogen level falls considerably while the FSH and LH values in the blood soar (as a reminder:

FSH is follicle-stimulating hormone; LH is the hormone that stimulates ovulation).[2]

The most notorious feature of this phase is hot flushes, which in addition to all the other unpleasant symptoms, can cause considerable discomfort and embarrassment. The night-time version of this is harmless from a physical point of view, but waking up soaking wet every night and having to change your sheets can be rather annoying. Other menopausal symptoms include mood changes, weight gain, joint pain, drier and thinner hair, increasingly wrinkly skin, increased forgetfulness and vaginal dryness.

## Menstrual cycle

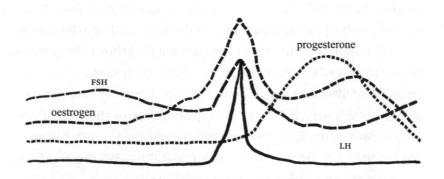

Release of hormones over one month; ovulation takes place when FSH peaks, followed by an increase in progesterone to allow the egg cells (if fertilised) to implant in the womb.

In this context I like to refer to my patient Iris, a vibrant woman around the age of fifty, who works as a visual artist and travels around the world to give presentations. She came to see me because she was regularly suffering from hot flushes, which were sometimes so bad she would walk off the stage soaking wet and with a red face. Her menopausal symptoms were severely impacting her daily life, and affected her sleep, so we decided to try out oestrogen therapy.

A month later she walked into my office a different woman. The hot flushes and soaked bedding were gone and she was sleeping well at night again. What's more, Iris reported that her libido had returned to the level it had been before her menopause.

Iris's case shows just how great an impact hormones can have on our physical and mental well-being.

Some people suffer during menopause more than others. Some women in the perimenopause have oestrogen levels lower than those of an adult man.[3] As the production of male hormones (in the adrenal glands and in the ovaries) often decreases less in women, their head hair may fall out and they may experience hair growth in typically male places, such as the chin and chest.[4] And although a woman remains post-menopausal for the rest of her life (that means to say that her oestrogen production ceases forever), these symptoms do reduce when a new hormonal balance is found. This process generally takes around five years, although it can sometimes take longer.

## The discovery of the menopause

The Bible tells the story of Abraham and Sarah: 'Abraham and Sarah were already old and well advanced in years, and Sarah was past the age of childbearing.' (Genesis 18:11) In the Netherlands, people often celebrate this new phase of life by placing dolls of these Biblical figures in their front gardens. The mention of the menopause in the Old Testament is one of the few references to the menopause from the premodern era. Despite her age, Sarah went on to give birth to a son. The parents named him Isaac – 'laughter' – supposedly after Sarah's reaction when she heard the happy news.

It's strange that books about medicine from the Middle Ages barely mention the menopausal transition. This is probably because life expectancy back then was lower, at around twenty-five or thirty, meaning that most women didn't reach the age of menopause onset. Aristotle was the first to report that female fertility has a time limit. In his *De partibus animalium* from 350 BC, the Greek philosopher and scientist states, probably inspired by the Ebers Papyrus, that women reach a reproductive limit around the age of forty-five. The Byzantine doctor Paul of Aegina confirmed this, but also referred to the influence of physique, stating that heavier women lose their menstrual cycles earlier, sometimes around the age of thirty-five. The *Trotula*, a set of three Italian books on women's conditions, treatments and aesthetics, written in the twelfth century by the female doctor Trota of Salerna, also mentions a critical moment for fertility, coming to the same conclusions as Paul of Aegina.[6]

Signs of perimenopause and reduced fertility in both men and women were referred to at that time as 'climacterium'. This term comes from Ancient Greek theories that a person's life is divided up into multiples of seven. These *climacteria* are 'critical periods' that, according to Greek philosophy and astrology, together form the ladder of life.[7] According to the Ancient Greeks, a phase of greater maturity and new responsibilities follows each successfully completed climacteric period. However, transitioning between stages is critical and ages divisible by seven entail more deaths.[8] Of all the transition phases, a number were known as the most dangerous – namely the age of forty-nine, followed by the switching point between late adulthood and early old age at sixty-three, with the 'annus climactericus maximum' in between: the age of fifty-six or 'androklas' (literally: man-killing).[9]

It was only at the start of the nineteenth century that the British royal and society physician Henry Halford drew attention to a climacteric 'disease'.[10] He had noticed that patients were often unwell for a period in middle age. Their 'vital forces' declined for a while, but later recovered. He suspected there was a disease that manifested itself at an older age but didn't follow the corresponding pattern of decline. For women, this climacteric disease occurred just before, after, or at the same time as their last menstruation. Shortly after this discovery, as is almost always the case when there is significant scientific interest, the phenomenon was given a name. In 1821, the French doctor Charles-Paul-Louis de Gardanne put forward the name 'la ménespausie', which in pseudo-Latin is derived from the Greek words for 'end' (*pausis*) and 'month' (*mèn*). He also coined the more controversial term *l'âge critique* for the ageing of men and woman.

## Golden years?

Our current impression of the menopause is a rather negative one. It mainly entails problems: you become infertile, cranky, fat, hairy and forgetful. Only one in five women don't experience any symptoms at all, but almost a third have so many symptoms that their work and social lives suffer.[11] The first negative reference to the menopause came from Galen (who further developed Hippocrates' ideas). Galen's 'humoral theory' was considered the standard in western medicine for centuries. According to this theory, in which everything revolves around balance, disease is caused by an imbalance of the four bodily fluids: phlegm, choler (yellow bile), black bile and blood. Galen believed these bodily fluids symbolised temperament and also determined your mood. Menstruation was seen as a natural way of removing any toxic substances from the body. According to this theory, the menopause leads to an internal accumulation of waste, which makes the woman hysterical. While doctors recommended therapies like bloodletting, 'hysterical old women' were often denounced as witches – with consequences.

This situation improved, to some extent, in the nineteenth century, when women ended up in psychiatric institutions as opposed to at the stake. But it was the obsession with the womb and associated sexuality in the prudish Victorian era that turned the menopause into a disease with psychiatric implications. While the French doctor Gardanne initially used the neutral term 'ménespausie' to refer to the menopausal transition, he later added 'the critical age of the woman' to the title of his book on this topic. The sex organs were seen as the new culprit for menopausal complaints (described as *hysteria*, a word derived from the Greek word for 'womb'), which is why the womb was often surgically removed at that stage. Even when the modern era of scientific innovations and technological progress dawned, negative opinions of the menopause remained. Whereas the Ancient Greeks spoke of an imbalance of the humors, researchers in the early twentieth century discovered that changes to hormones were the real cause of declining fertility.

Historically, the menopause was considered a natural transition; the introduction to a new phase of life that went hand in hand with greater wisdom and the ability to carry out more important tasks. It was often a desirable change for precisely that reason. Today, non-western population groups in particular focus on the positive aspects. The Japanese word for menopause is 'konenki', which means 'years of renewed energy'. In a

Dutch article (with the telling title 'The menopause is the road to death' – about Yvonne van den Hurk's show *Hormonologen*), reference is made to the Thai term 'thoi po ming', which means the 'golden years'.[12] In cultures in which menstruation is seen as impure, women are relieved when they reach 'the end of unclean days'.[13] Traditional tribes in Australia were at most amused when researchers asked them about symptoms of age-related sterility in women, for which they didn't even have a word.[14] Indigenous groups elsewhere in the world also view the menopause positively, with post-menopausal women regarded as sages, holding higher positions and enjoying greater social freedoms.[15]

Researchers believe it's possible that your own attitude towards the menopause influences how you experience this time.[16] While women in Asian countries suffer from few hot flushes or none at all, this is the main complaint among western women. In other cultures again, joint pain is the main symptom. But just as not all cultures with the same view of the menopause experience the same symptoms, it seems that multiple factors are at play here. Hormonal levels before the start of the menopause may also play a role. In certain groups and cultures, women breastfeed for longer, for example, which results in lower and more stable oestrogen levels during the perimenopause.[17] Lifestyle and body weight are also key factors when it comes to the pattern of symptoms. Eastern diets contain more phytoestrogens (see Chapter 2), which can affect the condition of your heart and blood vessels. Non-western women who live in cities often suffer more from insomnia and behavioural changes during the perimenopause than their family members who live in the countryside,[18] possibly because they're less active and are exposed to higher levels of toxic substances.

## Evolution and the grandmother hypothesis

*Homo erectus* differentiated itself from its predecessors as an upright species through its shorter arms and larger brain.[19] The latter adaptation proved crucial for its future. The larger skull meant that children were forced to be born earlier – otherwise they simply wouldn't fit through the birth canal – and were more dependent on their caregivers in the first stage of life.

Theories about the evolutionary benefits of the menopause relate to the evolution of early births. The role of the individual became less important and the role as a member of society more important, because more could be achieved together.[20] If you no longer have offspring in need of care, you can put more energy into bringing up other people's children. Female 'elders' fulfil an important role in the survival of the group. This was true in the past, but also today; just think of all the grand-parents who regularly babysit and give children chocolates and other treats 'for the journey'.

According to this 'grandmother hypothesis', the presence of grandmothers has an evolutionary advantage; fewer young children die and the mothers are more fertile because they don't need to use as much energy bringing up their children. As a result, they have more time to take care of their own supply of food. This phenomenon can also be observed in other animals. Orcas and short-finned pilot whales are the only other species that go through the menopause like humans, and in these animals, grandmothers are vitally important for the survival of the species.[21]

# Hormone therapies

You will no doubt recall Professor Brown-Séquard. His experiments with injections of sex hormones were soon replicated by others. Researchers also experimented with removing glands that produced sex hormones to cure certain diseases. We've known since ancient times that libido decreases in eunuchs – men whose testicles have been removed – but never before had specific interventions been made to the body's hormone production in order to reduce the disease burden. At the end of the nineteenth century, the Scottish army officer and doctor George Beatson suspected a link between female hormones and cancer.[22] He came up with this idea because farmers near Glasgow were removing the ovaries from their cows in order to guarantee a life-long production of milk. As the son of the personal physician of Queen Victoria, he was not afraid to experiment, so in 1899 he tried out this treatment in three women with metastatic breast cancer. And guess what? After removing their ovaries, the metastases of the tumour disappeared for a long time.

Beatson didn't receive the Nobel Prize for this discovery, but his Canadian colleague Charles Huggins was more fortunate later.[23] He applied the same principle and stopped the endogenous production of sex hormones in men with metastatic prostate cancer by removing the endocrine glands through castration. He too discovered that the metastases of these tumours temporarily receded following this intervention. So it's hardly surprising that from the 1960s onwards, when it became possible to produce sex hormones in larger quantities (firstly from animals and later synthetically), experiments were also carried out using female hormones to treat diseases.

In 1929, oestrogen was one of the first hormones to be discovered, in female urine. As women have measurably lower oestrogen levels after the menopause, the perimenopause was considered a 'state of deficiency'. From there it wasn't a big step towards treatment for menopausal symptoms. In the 1940s, the first substance came onto the market. It consisted of hormone extracts taken from the urine of pregnant mares and was given the name Premarin.

In his book *Feminine Forever*, which was published in 1963, the American gynaecologist Robert Wilson speaks of a 'menopause tragedy'.[24] The menopause was increasingly seen as a period of loss: a loss of youthfulness, vitality, femininity, hormones and, of course, fertility. Wilson referred to a mismatch between an increased life expectancy and an endocrine system unable to keep up with the rapid changes. But he believed it ought to be possible to help a post-menopausal woman with her ailments by giving her hormone supplements. Wilson's book was heavily romanticised; women started taking hormone pills en masse, which by then were made from the pulverised ovaries of horses and cows and later from synthetic oestrogens manufactured by the Dutch flagship of the pharmaceutical industry, Organon.

From the 1960s to the 1980s, the perimenopause was strongly medicalised. The menopausal transition shifted in people's minds from a natural and inevitable phenomenon to be endured to an illness that required medical attention. We now know that women who start menstruating before the age of eleven suffer more from symptoms of the perimenopause like hot flushes and migraines when they are older, and that these symptoms last longer.[25] The same applies to women who are overweight; the heavier you are, the more likely you are to suffer from hot flushes, joint pain and vaginal problems.[26] These are all symptoms that the doctors under the guidance of gynaecologist Wilson reportedly treated with oestrogen tablets. Despite increasing awareness of the side effects, these synthetic oestrogen variants became the most widely prescribed medications in the western world. Almost a quarter of all post-menopausal women used them over an extended period.[27]

Around the turn of the century, two major studies put an abrupt end to this. Although follow-up analyses and studies later showed that the risks associated with combined oestrogen and progesterone supplements were smaller than initially suggested by these trials, there still does appear to be a small increased risk of breast cancer and cardiovascular disease.[28,29] The question is whether this can outweigh the benefits, such as stronger bones and reduced risk of bowel cancer. Hormonal treatments do, however, work especially well in the short term for serious complaints, as was the case with my patient Iris, for whom the treatment proved very successful. When prescribing hormone treatment, most doctors now apply shared decision-making with their patients, counselling them on the risk-benefit ratio, after which the patient herself can decide. Doctors will also take into consideration other lifestyle factors which impact the risk of breast cancer, like alcohol consumption and obesity. If a doctor prescribes HRT they may recommend reducing alcohol consumption, for example, to offset the increased risk.

Hormones are also widely prescribed in alternative medicine. These include (but aren't limited to) food products rich in phytohormones, such as soya and red clover.[30] It's well-known that alcohol, red pepper, ginger tea and caffeine can trigger hot flushes, so avoiding these products can be another way to curb symptoms. Certain variants of our sex hormones such as DHEA (dehydroepianrosterone) are also recommended, although their effectiveness has not been scientifically proven and the long-term use of hormone treatments can also suppress your own production of hormones. In the alternative scene, animal hormones (such as thyreoidum, mentioned previously) are more common than in conventional medicine. Although their effectiveness is generally satisfactory, it is difficult to estimate the dosage because it is often unclear exactly how much of the hormone is contained in the capsules. In short, the discussion about whether 'natural' hormones should be combined with synthetic hormones, and if so, in which combination, is far from over.

## Hormones and how our memory works

The huge influence that sex hormones have on our lives is clear from the whole host of physical symptoms that can occur as soon as your hormone levels start to fluctuate. This influence also extends to the area of mental well-being; as mentioned earlier, sex hormones are involved in the development of the brain (see Chapters 3 and 4). Men seem to have a greater natural aptitude for spatial orientation, whereas women tend to have better verbal skills and long-term memory. In Chapter 7, we saw that women with stable hormone levels have a better memory as a result of the contraceptive pill,[31] and vice versa: fluctuations in hormone levels during the perimenopause lead to increased forgetfulness.[32] This phenomenon isn't only observed during pregnancy ('mumnesia' or 'baby brain') but also during the other major hormonal change in a woman's life. Memory problems during perimenopause are sometimes so severe that women fear they are starting to get dementia. While some people see an evolutionary benefit to 'pregnancy dementia' (your body is helping you focus on the most important task, namely caring for your unborn child), an evolutionary advantage to memory loss during the perimenopause is hard to find.

At the end of the 1940s, adult brain function was linked to female hormones for the first time. In a study into the endometrium, researchers noticed that treatment with oestrogens appeared to make participants more alert and improved their memory.[33] An American scientist decided to examine this unofficial finding in more detail and became the first to show that hormone therapy can improve the cognitive functions of post-menopausal women. This interesting, but still preliminary, finding came just at the right time for Robert Wilson, who keenly referred to it in his book *Feminine Forever*, thereby promoting both his book and the treatment.

It has since been repeatedly confirmed that a lack of oestrogen can, in fact, cause memory problems. An interesting example of this is in a 31-year-old American woman who unexpectedly experienced a decline in performance while training to become a pilot.[34] Doctors were puzzled for a long time, until they discovered that her hormone levels were indicative of early menopause. She made a full recovery after she started taking the contraceptive pill.

The oestrogens in the pill are known to protect a whole range of tissue cells, including those in the brain. They can even cause the grey matter, which contains the neurons, to increase in volume and hinder the accumulation of proteins (a symptom of Alzheimer's disease).[35] The hippocampus and frontal cortex, two areas of the brain that are primarily involved with memory, can produce sex hormones and help the maintenance of neurons.[36] Early menopause without the right hormonal supplementation could therefore increase the risk of memory disorders like Alzheimer's.

## Optimal timing of the female jubilee

With age-old attributions like 'great joy' and 'complete freedom, salvation and abundance', reaching the age of fifty – as with Abraham and Sarah – is traditionally seen as a special moment. In Biblical terms, it is a 'jubilee year': the year in which a field shouldn't be worked. And if the owner has had to rent it out to pay his debts, it should revert back to the rightful owner after another seven years have passed (the seven climacterics).[37]

A person's life expectancy has continually increased since the start of the twentieth century and puberty is commencing at an ever-younger age (see Chapter 3), but the age at which a woman reaches menopause, strangely enough, continues to hover around this magic number.[38] In ancient times, Aristotle and his followers reported that women usually had children up to the age of forty, some could still become mothers close to the age of fifty, but no cases were known after that age. Compared with other physiological functions of reproduction, menopause appears to have found an ideal point from which it rarely deviates. Evolutionary biologists in particular struggle to come up with an explanation for this phenomenon. If you base it on the principle of 'the more offspring, the greater the chance of survival of the species', it doesn't seem logical to put an end to it halfway through life. But the human population is still growing more rapidly than that of many other species, who have more offspring in relative terms. Scientific models suggest a type of 'optimal moment' for the menopause; until around the age of fifty, a woman's body can obviously still afford to get pregnant and bear children; after that, it is more beneficial to invest energy in ageing in a healthy way in order to be able to raise these children. Homo sapiens appears to favour quality over quantity, which ironically benefits the latter.

A modern-day sage who regularly emphasised the importance of timing was the Dutch footballing icon Johan Cruyff: 'There's only one moment you can be on time. If you're not there, you're either too early or too late.' Of course, he was talking about football, but this wisdom also applies to the menopause. As the timing of the menopause has remained the same for centuries, any deviations from this were seen as unhealthy. For a long time, menopause before the age of forty was known as POF: *premature ovarian failure*. The more neutral term *primary ovarian insufficiency* is now favoured, or the medical term 'climacterium praecox'. Whatever we call it, these women go through the menopause much earlier than is usually the case. In Europe, roughly one in a hundred thirty-somethings and in one in a thousand twenty-somethings go through the menopause. In most cases, the cause is unknown.[39]

In extreme cases, even children can go through the menopause. Take Amanda, for example: an eleven-year-old British girl who saw her weight double in the space of a few months and suffered from mood swings and hot flushes. Initially, doctors assumed these symptoms were caused by pubescent hormonal fluctuations. The diagnosis of a severely premature menopause was only made two years after her symptoms started. Amanda is the youngest post-menopausal female to have been reported.[40] Since she started taking hormone pills, which she will have to take until the age of fifty, she is doing much better, but if she ever wants to have children she will have to use an egg donor.

Besides being early, average or late, menopause can also come about naturally or unnaturally. As mentioned, a natural menopause is when you release your last few eggs, with the final egg leaving in your last period.[41] But you can also abruptly end up with an unnatural menopause – for example if the ovaries are rendered inoperative due to chemotherapy or an autoimmune disease, or if they are surgically removed. A famous example is the actress Angelina Jolie. She lost her mother to ovarian cancer and learned that she herself was carrying a mutation in the BRCA1 gene, which put her at increased risk of both ovarian and breast cancer.[42] Jolie therefore decided to have her ovaries and breasts surgically removed. She announced the news in a letter to the *New York Times*, which attracted so much attention that an 'Angelina Jolie effect' was observed in the healthcare system, with large numbers of women having tests for this gene or undergoing preventative surgery. Jolie spoke openly about suddenly going through the menopause, and although she had relatively few symptoms, she started hormone therapy – probably to retain her quality of life.

A number of years ago, it was assumed that the mother's age of menopause onset was a good predictor of when her daughter or daughters would go through the menopause.[43] The age that women have their first child has been increasing since the 1970s, which begs the question: is it possible to predict the moment at which fertility starts to decline? It was believed that if you wait too long, you might end up leaving it too late. Fortunately, there are now all sorts of technical and medical ways of extending a woman's fertility (such as freezing eggs, embryos and even ovaries – more about this later). These measures are, however, expensive and therefore not accessible to everyone.

In 2012, Danish researchers confirmed the long-held suspicion that around 50 per cent of the variability in menopausal age is attributable to genetics.[44] Identical twins have a menopausal age that is more similar than twins with different DNA.[45] At the same time, they shouldn't forget that around 50 per cent is *not* set out in our genetic blueprint, and that environmental and lifestyle factors can also influence this timing, which has evolutionary roots.

On an individual level, smoking – and even passive smoking – always comes up as the most important predictor of menopausal age.[46] The toxic substances in cigarettes – endocrine disruptors – cause an irreversible decline in both the quality and quantity of egg cells, which can cause perimenopause to begin up to four years sooner. Smoking can accelerate the drop in your oestrogen levels because the toxic substances in cigarette smoke impact your liver function, meaning that oestrogen is broken down more quickly. It's not surprising, then, that smoking causes so many fertility problems.

So why is research into how other endocrine disruptors influence the timing of the menopause so slow to get going? It's partly because of the long period of time between exposure and the development of symptoms. The Seveso disaster highlights this.[47] In 1976, there was an explosion in a chemical manufacturing plant in the Lombardy region of Italy, which suddenly exposed the young women of the population to the toxic chemical TCDD. (The Vietnam War had already proved how harmful TCDD is to human reproduction, when the US army used Agent Orange, which contains this dioxin, as part of its herbicidal warfare programme.) Around thirty years after the Seveso disaster, a group of researchers compared the menopausal age of women who lived near the chemical plant with that of women from other regions. They found that the greater a woman's exposure to the toxic substance, the younger she was when she had her final period.[48]

It was recently also discovered that the menopause can start earlier due to exposure to per- and polyfluorinated substances (PFAS), used for the non-stick layer in pans or for packaging and popular because of their stain-resistant and waterproof properties.[49] It will come as no surprise to the reader at this point in the book that a slower operation of the thyroid gland is also associated with increased exposure to both PFAS and TCDD.[50,51]

The effects of endocrine disruptors have been of interest to toxicologists and fertility experts for some time now. Future research will either confirm or disprove whether the frequent use of cosmetic products (which contain endocrine disruptors) can also lead to early menopause.[52]

## Contraception and menopause: from putting off to bowing out

Since its introduction in the 1960s, the contraceptive pill has led to a dramatic decrease in both the number of teen pregnancies as well as the number of unplanned pregnancies in Dutch women over the age of thirty-five.[53] Thanks to this family planning, Dutch women are having their first child at an ever-older age; this figure has risen from an average age of twenty-four in the decades after the Second World War to around thirty today. This trend towards 'putting off' can cause problems for women.

Ever since the pill solved the problem of contraception – *How do I* not *get pregnant?* – we have struggled with the issue of conception: *How do I* get *pregnant?* As already mentioned, the quantity and quality of egg cells dramatically decline with age. The contraceptive pill doesn't change that. Years before the menopause, fertility can decline so rapidly that a natural pregnancy becomes very unlikely. The disparity between biological and societal clocks has meant that the demand for medically assisted reproduction has increased significantly.

Around ten years after the arrival of the pill, technological feats like in-vitro fertilisation (IVF), whereby fertilisation of the egg takes place outside the body, increased opportunities for less fertile (and often older) couples. But with a success rate of just 20 per cent, this method didn't always lead to the desired result.[54] This is also because women often only considered IVF at a later age. In the late 1980s, 'cryopreservation' (from the Greek word for 'icy cold') offered a solution. With the help of this technique, biological material such as egg and sperm cells – or even fertilised embryos – can be frozen and stored for future use. In the same way our food keeps for longer if we store it in the freezer, lowering the temperature from 37 to –196 degrees Celsius causes the cells to go into hibernation, which keeps them young. This method can therefore be very useful to couples with anticipated fertility problems.

In the meantime, researchers have continued working on solutions for infertility in women who experience early menopause. In 2013, the new method of 'in-vitro activation' (IVA) was presented as a type of plug-in for IVF.[55] In this process, the less active ovaries of these young women are surgically removed and stimulated in a laboratory, which causes them to miraculously awaken from their sleep. Reimplantation of the activated tissue in combination with hormone stimulation therapy has already led to the birth of hundreds of healthy children all over the world.[56] In the Netherlands, this technique is currently only an option for women who experience early menopause, but it's becoming increasingly accessible to wealthy couples in the US who wish to decide for themselves when they want to start a family.

If younger egg and sperm cells offer so many advantages, and fertility treatments are increasing, you may wonder why we don't, as standard, freeze our egg and sperm cells when we're young. After all, there are currently no indications that test-tube babies or 'thawed' children develop less well than 'fresh' embryos.[57] The reason, besides the fact that it would considerably increase healthcare costs, is that a natural pregnancy is, to date, the most successful, not only in terms of the number of children, but also in terms of the health of the children and the mother. Our valiant attempts to imitate the complex hormonal plan via fertility treatments (together referred to as 'assisted reproductive technology') lead to striking hormonal peaks. Scientists are becoming increasingly fearful of the as-yet unknown consequences of this.

---

### Ice babies

In 1984, the world's first 'ice baby' was born in Australia. As an embryo, Zoe had spent two months in the freezer.[58] The cryopreservation technique was developed in order to reduce the number of multiple pregnancies in IVF and to minimise the associated risks. If you can store the embryos, you don't have to transfer them all at the same time and can choose an ideal moment to do so: when the mother has the most favourable hormone levels. A mother's eggs also don't have to be 'harvested'– a powerful stimulation using hormonal medication, with all the associated pain and risks – as often. All in all, cryopreservation offered a greater chance of pregnancy: by up to 65 per cent.[59]

That's a lot of benefits! After the seemingly unproblematic procedure with Zoe, many other 'ice queens' and 'ice kings' (or 'Eskimos', as they are sometimes called) soon followed. For a long time, this experimental technique was reserved for couples with a medical condition. After six hundred thousand successful births, this technique also became available commercially in 2012, which led to a huge rise in the number of treatments. The main reasons women cite as to why they decide to freeze their eggs are that they are still looking for the right partner or that starting a career is incompatible with starting a family. A number of large US companies, such as Facebook, Apple and Google, even offer their employees

---

financial support if they wish to carry out this expensive procedure.[60]

James Watson, who played a crucial role in the discovery of our DNA in 1953, was one of the first to criticise fertility technology. He didn't think embryo transplantations were a very good idea, to put it mildly, and four years before the first successful IVF procedure he predicted that 'all hell will break loose, politically and morally, all over the world'.[61] The new techniques were received somewhat more favourably than he predicted, but it's not inconceivable that exposure to high concentrations of hormones could have long-term consequences. An example of this was already mentioned in the Introduction, whereby the side effects of DES, an oestrogen preparation that was mainly prescribed to prevent miscarriages in the Netherlands before the 1970s, were more drastic than expected for the mothers as well as their children and even grandchildren.

With fertility treatments, synthetic antioestrogens are used to promote follicle growth, after which FSH induces 'superovulation'. In its guidelines, the Dutch Society of Obstetrics and Gynaecology also lists other hormone treatments, such as progesterone or the pregnancy hormone hCG, corticosteroids or substances that stimulate ovulation.[62] The huge range of hormone treatments for fertility can be very confusing (not just for the body), and because these treatments are relatively new, possible long-term effects, including those for future generations, can't be ruled out.

This uncertainty around long-term effects leaves room for speculation. It has been claimed, for example, that children conceived via a test tube could be at increased risk of autism-like disorders. However, a large-scale Swedish study carried out in 2013 rejected this claim.[63] It's more likely that specific characteristics of those parents who undergo fertility treatment (such as an older age, health problems and more frequent multiple births) have a greater influence on the health of their children than the treatment itself.[64]

With all the statistics about success rates with fertility issues, these procedures can still seem like a lottery, except that we likely have a considerable influence on the outcome. This is because our own hormones are key when it comes to the success of fertility treatment. In short, if you have reduced fertility you should schedule the embryo transfer for spring, and you'd do well to lay off the coffee for a while. Research has shown that exposure to springtime light activates cells that stimulate the release of LH and FSH: two hormones that are important for egg cell maturation and ovulation. Spring is the winner when it comes to the likelihood of getting pregnant after fertility treatment. Caffeine, on the other hand, has a negative effect: drinking more than five cups of coffee a day is just as disastrous as smoking cigarettes when it comes to the likelihood of a successful IVF attempt.[65]

## Pregnant with your own granddaughter

As well as providing solutions to fertility problems, technological progress and knowledge can also lead to ethical and societal dilemmas, as James Watson predicted. Thanks to synthetic hormones, cryopreservation and IVF and IVA techniques, it's now possible to get pregnant even after the menopause: by fertilising premenopausal eggs and transferring them, if necessary, to a surrogate mother. In 1999, a 66-year-old British woman became the oldest woman to give birth to her own grandchildren, after her son and his partner struggled to carry babies to term. The honour of the oldest mother, however, ever goes to Omkali Charan Singh from India. She and her husband had only daughters, who were unable to inherit any possessions due to their sex. At the (estimated) age of seventy-four, she therefore desperately attempted to have a son via IVF.[66] And it was successful!

In the Netherlands this is prohibited by law; for many years, the maximum age for these procedures was forty-five in order to protect the health of both mother and child. As the strict criteria often pushed women to go abroad for these procedures, and because life expectancy has increased, the maximum age was recently increased to forty-nine. Experts suspect post-menopausal pregnant women won't be an un-usual sight in a few years' time.

Another scenario that no one had considered when medi-cal assistance for fertility issues was in its infancy was the way unborn children can experience time travel. An example of this is the Chinese boy Tiantian, who was born with the help of a surrogate mother in Laos in 2018, four years after both of his parents died in a car crash.[67] As the surrogate mother didn't give birth in China, his grandparents fought for Tiantian to be granted Chinese citizenship.[68] Emma, another such example, is only actually one year younger than her surrogate mother. During a round of IVF twenty-four years earlier, her biological parents had a number of embryos frozen, not all of which were transferred.[69] When they donated the remaining cells to a young couple, a successful pregnancy caused a bizarre journey through time.

Slowly but surely, attention is shifting from outstanding technical features of hormonal treatments to ethical dilemmas: how far can we take this? Could a woman, one day, get pregnant with her frozen brother or sister?

# ADAM and the andropause

So far, the 'male menopause' has generally remained out of the spotlight, probably because it is a much more gradual process. But it's long been known that men also experience changes during this period of transition. The German neurologist Kurt Mendel (1874–1946) borrowed the term 'climacterium' from the Ancient Greeks to describe symptoms such as lethargy, loss of strength, attacks resembling hot flushes and emotional instability in ageing men: *climacterium virile*.[70] He couldn't fully explain it, but his research was still extremely important. In his systematic search for possible causes of these symptoms, he stumbled upon the products of the gonads before these hormones were discovered. He assumed that these substances were responsible for sex-specific characteristics, and that a decrease in these substances would therefore make a woman more masculine and a man more feminine, relatively speaking.

Not much later, the English gynaecologist Robert Barnes made a strong statement in response to Mendel's comments about the climacterium virile: he stated that the andropause is in no way similar to the complete revolution the female body experiences when the hormonal deterioration of the ovaries begins. By advancing the term 'menopause', the male half of the world's population has been excluded from the hormonal midlife crisis for the past century. Attention has mainly been focused on the abrupt changes to the female body, with the consequence that male symptoms of this period of transition have been virtually forgotten.

It's true that women experience more hormonal changes than men. As there's no abrupt moment of transition in men as there is with menopause, Barnes appears to be right; men often experience fewer effects of the hormonal ageing process and their symptoms arise more gradually. The main male hormone, testosterone, doesn't fluctuate monthly and its production doesn't stop abruptly like the production of oestrogen in women. Instead, it gradually decreases by 1 per cent each year from the age of thirty. In the 2016 book *How Men Age*,[71] the American medical anthropologist Richard Bribiescas lists the biological and social advantages of the andropause caused by lower and more stable testosterone levels: more fat deposits (better chance of survival during famines), less reckless behaviour and greater knowledge of social group processes.

Thanks to the work of Mendel and the discovery of many hormones shortly afterwards, there has been continued interest in hormonal changes as we age.[72] With our current knowledge, we can respond to complaints about the transition years in a more focused manner. We now know that testosterone levels start to fluctuate on a daily basis in men over the age of forty, after which they gradually decrease to around 70 per cent of the normal level by the age of eighty.[73] The term 'andropause' has therefore been replaced by the more appropriate term 'androgen deficiency in the ageing male', abbreviated to ADAM.[74] Due to the functions of testosterone, a shortage of androgens can, as Mendel observed, lead to a lower libido, decreased muscle mass, fewer red blood cells, weaker bones and a gloomier mood – an obvious parallel to the loss of female hormone.

The memoirs of the Dutch doctor and writer Ivan Wolffers highlight the impact of these types of changes. He was diagnosed with prostate cancer in 2002. As testosterone sends a growth signal to prostate cells and can therefore trigger (metastatic) cancerous cells to grow, he was 'chemically castrated' by means of hormone-blocking substances – a less invasive procedure than full castration, for which Charles Huggins won his Nobel Prize. In his book *Heimwee naar de lust*, whose title, '*A Longing for Lust*' refers to what the author regards as one of the most unpleasant side effects of hormone therapy, Wolffers shows that a dry summary of symptoms falls short of the actual experiences of patients.[75] He also explains how rapidly he noticed himself changing from the tough, self-confident man he had always been to a 'soft, hairless eunuch [and] impotent cry-baby', who was hypersensitive and seriously questioned 'where [he] began and the hormones ended'.

His book provides a useful insight into physical changes, such as loss of muscle mass and hair, but also into the consequences for mental health and personality. Wolffers also suffered from hot flushes as a result of the treatment. Though we associate hot flushes with post-menopausal women, they're not unusual for men with ADAM either. It's not yet clear what exactly causes hot flushes, but researchers think sex hormones might affect the centres in your brain responsible for temperature regulation. The case of a 32-year-old British soldier is particularly striking. He lost both testicles in an accident in Afghanistan and ended up in a 'traumatic andropause'.[76] In the first few weeks, his body temperature fluctuated, apparently without reason, and doctors tried to treat the symptoms with antibiotics. It was only after intramuscular injections with testosterone that his temperature stabilised, which proves just how important (male) hormones are for everyday bodily functions.

# Testosterone for eternal youth?

It is estimated that only one in every fifty men who believe they suffer from ADAM actually has a shortage of male hormone.[77] That's why treatment with testosterone is generally not the most appropriate solution. Despite this, the substance is more popular than ever; over the past ten years, the sale of testosterone preparations has increased fivefold. In the nineteenth century, Brown-Séquard and his followers announced that they had 'rejuvenated' themselves with injections containing animal testicular extract. We now know that this was a placebo effect, but the neurologist's enthusiasm led to global interest in what was reputedly a key to eternal youth, with many daring doctors experimenting with testicular extracts or even with transplantation of the organ. After the discovery of testosterone, hormone therapy – in parallel with oestrogen supplementation for women – became extremely popular for a long time.

The supplementation of decreasing hormone levels in men hadn't yet been proved a good idea. For example, a recent paper showed that topping up testosterone did not have any beneficial effects on bone fractures, and even increased fracture incidence for those individuals.[78] Yet, the masses believed in it and this belief was bolstered by books like *The Male Hormone* by the American microbiologist Paul de Kruif.[79] In this book, which was published in 1945 and inspired by scientific experiments with the recently discovered testosterone, he praises the 'magical' substance, which he believes is essential for the golden older years ('when life is richest and its demands the heaviest'). He believed that many success stories would ensue. Despite the lack of scientific evidence for the theory that testosterone fulfils its promises, the number of low-testosterone clinics (or 'low-T' clinics) where people can go for a rejuvenating formula is on the rise.[80]

It may be the case that the restorative effect of a testosterone boost is due to an increase in red blood cells.[81] Testosterone stimulates the kidneys to produce more EPO, a glycoprotein hormone naturally produced by the peritubular cells of the kidney, which (as we also know from various doping scandals) helps transport oxygen to body tissue more quickly. Of course, this benefits your endurance and overall condition, but it doesn't mean that you actually get any younger. One side effect of testosterone injections is that the body retains more salt and water thanks to ADH (antidiuretic hormone or vasopressin), which can cause an increase in blood pressure. In general, men have a lower life expectancy than women, and testosterone supplementation further reduces this.[82] Studies with eunuchs have repeatedly shown that they live up to twenty years longer than their uncastrated counterparts.[83] For the time being, testosterone is therefore not the end point in the search for the elixir of life.

The exceptionally high number of age-related ailments in young body builders is also inconsistent with the belief that an extra dash of testosterone increases vitality.[84] But that 'dash' is key: the amount used for sporting purposes is many times greater than the amount needed to supplement the body's own production.[85] And even if you were to limit yourself to that small amount, it would still not solve symptoms of the andropause in a middle-aged man. This is because a low level of testosterone is sometimes not the cause, but the result, of deteriorating health. This makes the approach for treating this type of complaint especially complicated.

With weight gain, for example, the body fat of an overweight man converts testosterone into the female oestrogen.[86] One of the first symptoms of a low testosterone level is a decreased sexual desire, as Wolffers describes so well. The America and UK of the 1940s used that knowledge to give young homosexual

227

men a controversial and experimental 'treatment' with testosterone preparations. It was long believed that their 'female constitution' could be 'rectified' by immersing them in male hormone.[87] We don't know whether their libido increased, but the anticipated change in sexual orientation certainly did not take place.

All in all, the decrease in testosterone levels in middle-aged men is part of a natural process that has been going on for thousands of years, and which appears to predominantly have biological and sociological advantages, as Richard Bribiescas describes. Despite all the success stories, treatment with testosterone can't indefinitely hold off the decline of the young, athletic, male body. That's why the healthiest conclusion at this point is that it's more effective for middle-aged men to improve and maintain a healthy lifestyle than to go grasping at straws with a daily dose of testosterone. Ultimately, Mother Nature is fair and gives both women and men, in the menopause or andropause, a nudge towards the next phase of life.

# 9

# A New Balance

*After a Hormone-filled Life*

At the start of the 1990s, the American relationship counsellor and author John Gray achieved global success with his book *Men Are from Mars, Women Are from Venus*.[1] By highlighting recognisable aspects of both sexes and linking these to day-to-day examples and explanations, he tapped in to something we are all curious about: the fundamental differences between men and women. In nature, it is generally accepted that these differences exist. During a trip to a children's farm we learn that a colourful peacock is the male and a plainer specimen the female. Compared with animals, the difference between the human sexes doesn't seem as distinct, but appearances can be deceptive, as there are numerous sex-specific differences in appearance, build, organ function and even in the way in which men and women get ill, recover and age. Our hormones – of course – play a key role in this.

Whether we are male or female depends on a single biological difference: the presence or absence of the Y chromosome in our genetic makeup, which consists of a total of forty-six building blocks. The information on this male chromosome is responsible for the development of testicles and therefore the production of testosterone (see also Chapter 2), which shapes the male body for the rest of life. Even before birth, the sex hormones ensure that the physical structure develops differently in men and women.

In general, men are taller and have a different skull shape (and therefore a different face) to women. As women are designed to be able to give birth to a child, they generally have wider hips. With the stereotypical female hourglass figure, the navel is under the waist, whereas with the male V-shape (with broader shoulders than hips), the navel is above the narrowest point. We also differ in terms of fat distribution: men store surplus energy in the belly, whereas this is generally stored around the hips and thighs in women.[2] If you look carefully, you even notice that flat feet are more common in older men than in older women.[3] In turn, women blink more often than men, and the frequency with which they do so increases with age.[4]

There aren't only external differences – we are different on the inside too. Not only are the thyroid, liver and kidneys smaller in women, but the brain, heart, lungs and oesophagus are also significantly larger in men. Why is it important to know this as you age? Because knowledge of the differences between the male and female body is crucial when it comes to providing appropriate medical care. It was only recently discovered that many age-related ailments progress differently in men and women and that changes to sex hormones promote this. In short, ageing is a broad term; 'senior' means 'older person' as well as 'more experienced'. The experience of ageing is just as individual as the senior-citizen discount on public transport is universal. One person may still be full of vitality, even in sexual terms, while another is afraid of getting sick and yet another has already started deteriorating due to ill health. In this chapter I will show what happens physically between the ages of sixty and seventy-five. In this phase of life, the body experiences a hormonal U-turn, through which it prepares itself for old age. What's fascinating is that men and women start to become more similar in hormonal terms.

## Changing of the hormonal guard

Biological sex is one of the first distinctions we make, often subconsciously, for ourselves and others. You are either a man or a woman – even though these categories are increasingly experienced differently. There are all sorts of ingrained stereotypical assumptions attached to that distinction: girls cry more than boys, adolescent boys don't talk, the study of psychology is for women and the man of the house repairs the kitchen cupboards. And while research has shown that women cause fewer traffic accidents than men, we always hear about their inability to park.[5]

When they hear the word 'hormones', most people instantly think of all the differences between men and women. And many of these differences *are* caused by sex hormones. However, something unusual happens in old age. As we age, the hormonal differences between men and women slowly dissipate. Despite the fact that oestrogen drops abruptly in post-menopausal women, whereas testosterone falls gradually in ageing men, there are similarities between the sexes in biochemical terms. While oestrogens are in power in women from puberty onwards, a change of the hormonal guard takes place at around the age of sixty: testosterone originating from the ovaries and adrenal glands begins to take charge. In most older men, androgens maintain a narrow majority, but compared with younger men, they suddenly have up to three times as much oestrogen.[6] If you are already overweight as an elderly man, you gain even more weight because the fat tissue itself also produces oestradiol, a form of oestrogen, from testosterone.

After a life of hormonal and other physical differences, men and women start to become more alike in this phase of life, which some married couples emphasise by sporting matching waterproofs and hairstyles. The hormonal shift is reflected in the way in which the older body adapts physically. In women, changes to hair, skin, voice and behaviour are somewhat more noticeable than in men. Let's take a closer look at these conspicuous features, starting with body hair.

In many people, the ageing process results in hair *loss*: men lose hair on their legs, chest, arms and head. Meanwhile, an altered hormonal balance can lead to hair *growth* in older women. This increase in body hair, brought about by testosterone, is mainly seen on body parts where men typically experience hair growth: the chin and the upper lip. This phenomenon is also known as 'hirsutism'. Even though testosterone levels in older women remain lower than that of their male peers, they experience significantly more problems with facial hair growth – and baldness – in comparison with younger women.[7] The fact we don't encounter women with beards on a weekly basis is more down to the dominant beauty ideal (and the opportunities to remove unwanted hair growth through epilation and laser removal) than a lack of hormonal effort.

---

### Hair = power

Physical and spiritual power have been attributed to body hair for many years, long before testosterone's role in this

---

was discovered. Just think of Samson from the Bible, whose strength resided in his long hair. And if you know your saints, think of Saint Wilgefortis, also known as Uncumber.[8] She had firmly decided to dedicate her life to God, but her father – the king of Portugal – had other plans and sought a husband for her. Her prayers to 'unencumber' herself from both men were answered: Wilgefortis grew an unattractive beard that gave her an even more powerful appearance. Unfortunately for Wilgefortis, her beard was seen as a sign of the devil and she was crucified. Her story resembles that of the first female Pope Joan, who may also have suffered from adrenogenital syndrome.[9] In later times, women accused of witchcraft had their heads shaved prior to their trials to do away with any unseen forces.

Men attach great importance to their hair. The Kenyan Masai, for example, are convinced that the loss of facial hair in their chiefs goes hand in hand with a loss of leadership qualities; at various stages of life, the women would shave the men's heads (for example, when they get married or when they reach the age of an elderly wise man).[10] You might think this knowledge even made it as far as the White House, where the former president Trump did his utmost to maintain his blonde coiffure so as to demonstrate his vitality and power. He reportedly still takes finasteride for this on a daily basis,[11] which hinders the breakdown of testosterone and therefore also suppresses hair loss. His personal physician doesn't reveal whether the former president also suffers from the common side effects of this, which include loss of libido, impotence and growth of mammary glands. But as long as his hair looks good ...

## Skin and bone structure

Besides hair loss or growth, skin also changes as we age. Whereas cosmetic treatments and hormonal remedies based on testosterone (such as finasteride) sometimes make it difficult to estimate a person's age based on their hairdo alone, our skin appears to be a better predictor, especially for women.[12]

Wrinkles can give such an accurate impression that researchers train computer systems to estimate the age of fugitives on this basis.[13] Of course, not smoking and avoiding alcohol also help, as do healthy sleep, using a good night cream from a young age (without complicated additives) and protecting yourself from the sun when outside. However, hormones also play a role in the deterioration of the skin. The oestrogens that give a woman smoother and younger-looking skin than a man for most of her life let her down relatively abruptly after the menopause.[14] Her skin becomes wrinkly and loses elasticity and robustness; wounds also heal less quickly.[15]

The assumption that men age more attractively than women, with men like George Clooney, Pierce Brosnan and Richard Gere as examples, appears to be based on rising oestrogen levels in ageing men. On the other hand, this can also cause men to gain weight (the so-called 'dad bod').[16]

Whereas a decrease in oestrogen levels mainly affects the skin, the shape of the face of older women appears to change under the influence of testosterone, which is now dominant.[17] In particular, this affects the ratio between the length and width of the face. The higher the testosterone level, the wider the face becomes related to the length. For boys in puberty, this leads to the formation of an adult face,[18] but women with PCOS also notice similar changes to their facial structure.[19] Broader jawlines and more prominent eyebrows are sometimes also observed in female bodybuilders who increase their androgen levels through the use of steroids.[20,21]

Testosterone is not the only factor, however. In this phase, we not only observe changes to the skin, facial structure and hair of ageing women, but also to their personality.

## Male and female roles

By losing its task of reproduction, it seems that the female body goes through a role reversal and expresses its power in a different way. Research carried out by the American scientists Margaret Zube and Esther Perelman, experts in the field of relationship issues in older people, showed that older men tend to become more introspective, whereas women are more likely to take on new projects and to raise their profile outside family life.[22]

A man not only becomes gentler as he ages, but also somewhat gloomier. He is more likely to feel downcast than in his younger days. On this psychosocial level too, men and women become more similar. Women have a higher risk of affective disorders such as depression throughout their lives. This is related to the quantity of monoamines: hormone-like signalling substances in the brain that play a role in emotions and resemble neurotransmitters like dopamine and serotonin.[23] In healthy, adult women, those monoamines are erratic; the cyclical variations to their sex hormones are, in part, responsible for fluctuations that make women more susceptible to depression. But the change in sex hormones as a woman ages causes steroids to appear on the scene, which appear to have a beneficial effect on monoamines in women. Ultimately, the risk profiles become even more extreme; research shows that 86 per cent of all suicides in older people are committed by men.[24] Due to the complex nature of depression and the factors involved in suicide, the exact role that our hormones play in this is, of course, difficult to establish.

Broader jawlines can also benefit women in their work. A more masculine look is often associated with dominance and success. Research shows that CEOs of international companies and leaders of major organisations tend to have broader jawlines, relatively speaking.[25] Evidently we think of people with broader jawlines as more competent. In electoral campaigns, the appearance of the top candidate is also crucial. It takes only a fraction of a second for voters to form an impression of someone's competence,[26] which seems to be the decisive factor when we walk into the polling station, overloaded with information. In an experiment, children between the ages of five and thirteen were shown photos of electoral candidates and asked: who would you choose as the captain of your boat? Here too, those with broader jawlines were favoured,[27] and these children were able to predict the electoral result with relative success.

Let's return to the behavioural changes in people as they approach retirement age. Many a management guru is aware of the sex-specific change to the behaviour of older employees.[28] As they age, male employees care less for hierarchy and become more personal and human. Women are more likely to become rationally motivated as opposed to emotionally motivated. Although these are generalisations, this knowledge helps us better understand group dynamics and therefore better manage older employees.

# The ageing voice

Finally, old age sometimes gives itself away even if we can't see the person in question. This is because your voice also changes as you age. Men's voices usually gradually get higher, whereas women's voices deepen.[29] For female professional singers, this 'post-menopausal voice syndrome' can be problematic for their careers.[30] Women are often familiar with the effect that their monthly cycle can have on the pitch of their voice.[31] Many singers have therefore learned to schedule their work according to their menstrual cycle, or they take hormonal contraceptives to protect the quality of their voice. On the other hand, the higher pitch of a man's voice may indicate that his fertility is coming to an end. From an evolutionary point of view, a deeper voice is an effective way of attracting female interest. Scientific research confirms that women are more attracted to men with deeper voices – especially when they are at their most fertile.[32] In addition, men appear to change their voice based on the (presumed) social hierarchy between them and their conversation partner; if this is another man with whom he is competing for the attention of a potential partner, his voice will deepen.[33] An ageing man, with changed interests and lower levels of testosterone, therefore loses the lower notes – as he no longer needs to reproduce.[34]

As you can see, there is plenty of evidence that men and women become more similar as they age. However, sex-specific characteristics continue to exist. You can count the number of knitting grandads on one hand, for example. The fact that the body is controlled by a female or male cocktail of signalling substances for an entire lifetime certainly leaves its mark.

## Different symptoms of the same condition

First of all, general anatomical differences between the male and female body can explain why one sex is more susceptible to a certain condition than the other. For older people this difference becomes even more apparent, for example with cystitis.

After the menopause, women become more susceptible to this than they were previously, because the thickness of the lining of the urethra decreases when the oestrogen level in their blood drops.[35] For men, the number of urinary tract infections remains relatively constant throughout adulthood. The anatomical reason for this is that a woman's urethra is straight and short (just four centimetres long), whereas that of a man is on average twenty-two centimetres long and curved.[36] Only an extremely determined pathogen can therefore reach the male bladder. However, as the prostate grows over time, bladder infections become more common in older men. Often, such an infection requires more intensive treatment than before, to ensure that it doesn't lead to pyelitis or sepsis.

There are differences relating to the skeleton too; male bones are generally stronger. Older women, on the other hand, are more likely to suffer from collapsed vertebrae and arthritis in the knee.[37] This is also related to the shape of the female pelvis, which is positioned in such a way that a mild form of knock-knees is more common in women. The knee joints are therefore under greater pressure throughout a woman's life, which causes them to wear out more quickly than a man's.[38] It might seem unfair, but it's true: because worn-out knee joints can make you less mobile more quickly as a woman, you are more susceptible to conditions caused by a lack of movement and obesity, which in turn increases the likelihood of adult-onset diabetes.

Men also have better alcohol tolerance, which means they can stay sober for longer. A woman's liver is not only smaller, but also produces less alcohol dehydrogenase, which is the group of enzymes that accelerates the breakdown of alcohol. After the same glass of wine, more alcohol is left in a woman's blood than a man's.[39] As women generally have relatively more body fat, alcohol is also excreted less quickly, and they become tipsy more quickly.

Do women always draw the short straw as a result of these differences in metabolism? Not always. In some cases, they benefit. Because they metabolise fat more effectively, for example, women can store more energy in the form of sugar, which means they naturally have a greater endurance.[40] Despite the fact that, in relative terms, men have more muscle mass, a bigger heart, a greater lung capacity and a greater capacity for the transportation of oxygen, they are no match for the more energy-efficient women on a long bike ride.[41]

Incidentally, these are just a few examples of demonstrable differences between the male and female body. But until recently, this knowledge was rarely applied to the treatment of conditions, and this has put individual patients at risk. The differences between our bodies and how they behave is crucial, not only in terms of recognising symptoms, but also in terms of determining the best course of treatment. It was recently discovered, for example, that cardiovascular disorders present themselves differently in women and men. Chest pain (the well-known sign of an impending heart attack) usually radiates to the left arm or the jaw in men, whereas women usually experience pain in their back or neck – and sometimes they don't experience any pain at all.[42] The perceived atypical nature of their complaints (such as dizziness and fatigue) means that female patients *and* their doctors often fail to recognise signs of an impending heart attack.[43] 'The woman's heart is coveted, but also gravely misunderstood,' cardiologist Janneke Wittekoek writes in her book *Het vrouwenhart* ('*The Woman's Heart*').[44] The cardiologist and professor Angela Maas brought global attention to the female heart with her research into the differences between men and (post-menopausal) women in terms of the risk of cardiovascular disease and its treatment.

The fact that diseases also behave sex-specifically makes it especially complicated when it comes to recognising symptoms. In the case of coronary artery calcification in women, the smaller arteries constrict over their whole length, whereas in men, constrictions in the larger vessels of the heart are more localised but also more serious.[45] Female former smokers are more likely to have a heart attack than non-smokers for a good fourteen years after their last cigarette, whereas the effect of smoking disappears in men within eight years of their last cigarette.[46]

Even if we use tried-and-tested technology, a suspected heart attack is still more difficult to prove in women than men. An electrocardiogram (ECG), for example, is considerably less reliable for a woman due to the different shape of her chest.[47] Better detection methods are possible, but these are often more expensive and less user-friendly. That's why an ECG is still considered the gold standard for the diagnosis of a heart attack. Another important objection to the ECG is that this technology, just like many medications, was developed on the basis of research using male test subjects. The cardiologist Angela Maas explains: 'The man was the norm; heart complaints in women were vaguer and were dismissed by male doctors as either symptoms of the menopause or as whingeing.'

The assumption that the man is the norm can also be observed when it comes to screening for bowel cancer, the most common cancer in women after breast cancer. The procedure relies on detecting miniscule quantities of blood in faeces but this doesn't appear to be a good indicator in women. Not only is the tumour of the bowel often in a different location – in women it's usually at the right of the stomach, where it can't be examined as easily, whereas in men it is usually on the left – but the passage of the contents of the gut is slower in women.[48] This means that more blood can be reabsorbed into the bowel, as a result of which it doesn't end up in the faeces, where it would be possible to detect it using the available screening test.

---

## Bikini medicine

If a woman's body functions so differently from a man's body, why has the female physiology been considered a 'light version' of the male body for so long? The answer is simple but crude: since the emergence of modern medicine, a lot more research has been carried out on men than women.

According to Marek Glezerman, an Israeli emeritus professor of obstetrics and gynaecology and author of the book *Gender Medicine* ('Ook getest op vrouwen'),[49] first published in 2016, the dramatic results of medical studies carried out on pregnant women in the 1950s and 1960s played an important role in this. When it was established that the children of the participants displayed abnormalities, the American Food and Drug Administration (FDA) deemed that reason enough to prohibit certain forms of medical research being carried out on women of fertile age. Men are the preferred choice when it comes to testing medicines because they don't have a menstrual cycle, so their hormone levels are much more stable. As sex hormones can influence the metabolism of drugs, however, this exclusion led to a considerable shortfall in knowledge of how illness presents in women and an associated lack of knowledge about treatment with medication.

This shortfall is so great that it takes much longer for women to receive a diagnosis from a doctor, and they often

---

end up with the wrong diagnosis.[50] Research from Oxford University suggests that not only is medication prescribed later for women than men, but also that medication, such as that used to treat heart failure, would have to be prescribed in different dosages for women in order to be effective.[51] Experts in the field of biological differences between the sexes refer to this as 'bikini medicine': a dangerous blind spot that arises from the long-held assumption that women only differ from men in the places hidden by a bikini.[52] The result of this is that women live in poorer health for longer than necessary.

Is the solution, then, to simply carry out more scientific research on women, to fill the gaps? Glezerman and his colleagues call – and rightly so – for a more in-depth analysis of the *differences* between the sexes. These differences, they assume, developed as a result of diverging physical demands many centuries ago. Our distant ancestors divided up day-to-day tasks in order to increase the chance of survival. Put simply, the women's task was to reproduce and give birth, for which they needed enough stability and energy stores in their lower body. Men went out hunting and developed a talent for spatial awareness.[53] The fact that we have mainly moved away from these roles in today's society doesn't mean that the physiological differences have suddenly disappeared. Glezerman and his colleagues are committed to enriching medical knowledge through sex-specific research and teaching. They expect that the ensuing improvements to medical healthcare will save lives. The hope is that the emancipation of women in the twenty-first century will also extend to medical healthcare so that women too will get an approach and treatment tailored to *their* body.

Being aware of the differences between the sexes is absolutely vital when it comes to cardiovascular disease. Despite the fact we've known about the different course of the disease for men and women since the 1990s (known as 'Yentl syndrome' – as depicted in the 1983 Barbra Streisand movie of the same name),[54] we are only really starting to pay attention to this difference now, thirty years later. In its recent campaigns, the Dutch Heart Foundation decided to focus specifically on cardiovascular disease in women.

# Winter body

The shift in the role of sex hormones in the bodies of older people also affects other endocrine systems. One such 'affected hormone' is the thyroid hormone. The declining production of sex hormones leads to less effective thyroid hormone receptors, which in turn means that thyroid hormone is less able to fulfil its role. As a result, processes in the energy system slow down and fat tissue increases.[55] That excess fat tissue produces less leptin due to a decline in sex hormones. This satiety hormone (see Chapter 5) ensures an appropriate supply of energy during adulthood. Leptin influences your eating behaviour so that you stop eating when you're sufficiently nourished. In practical terms, it prevents you from eating until you burst and storing that surplus energy as fat. The system is wonderfully designed; if your reserves are too low, your fat percentage decreases, as does your leptin level, which increases your desire to eat.

But the ageing body can become resistant to leptin,[56] similar to how it can become resistant to insulin in the case of diabetes. As a result, you don't get that feeling of satiety and your body is encouraged to eat more. Compared with the sex hormones, leptin plays only a supporting role as you age, but we shouldn't underestimate its influence. When researchers gave mice a small quantity of additional leptin, the animals lost up to 40 per cent of their body weight.[57] Despite the fact that fat mass is the main producer of leptin, the release of the hormone is mainly controlled by the sex hormones.[58]

In the autumn and winter our metabolism slows down, which causes us to gain weight – this is why we temporarily develop a 'winter body'. In older people, the shifted production of hormones results in more physical changes. In general, people gain weight as they age; fat mass increases and muscle mass decreases.[59] This makes it especially difficult for older people to maintain a slim figure. It's just a matter of time before their winter body becomes a year-round body. But it is increasingly important to stay fit as we age. Your muscle mass percentage is a good indicator of how many years you have left: the higher the percentage, the longer your life expectancy.[60] Both men and women benefit from physical activity as they age if they want to prevent muscle loss.

## Old is the new young

Like in other life phases, major hormonal changes clearly accompany incipient old age. And while men and women become more alike in that respect, these changes unfold in different ways. For both sexes, endocrine problems present themselves rather atypically in old age, and not always as described in medical textbooks. And while we collectively appear to fear old age, we each experience the changes in our body differently. On birthdays we only admit how 'young' we are when cajoled into doing so. We associate old age with decline because our body functions less effectively. We suddenly can't hear as well, run as fast – or run at all – or learn as quickly as before. Everyone wants to *become* old, but no one wants to *be* old.

As part of the ageing process of the human body, the endocrine system faces a similar downwards spiral; most hormonal, signalling chemicals decrease.[62] But if you study the ageing of the endocrine system more closely, you will notice that these changes are *adjustments* that contribute to your health as opposed to hindering it. In order to understand how 'old is the new young', we need the biological terms 'homeostasis' and 'feedback'. Our body has the ability to continually monitor our health. It ensures that the inner environment can recover and remain in balance even when conditions change. This physiological process is referred to as homeostasis. If the hormonal balance fluctuates, there is a problem. If, for example, your insulin and blood sugar levels are 'too high', this could be a symptom of a pancreatic disorder, which may result in insulin resistance. In that case, older people are treated with medications or synthetic hormone preparations to stabilise these levels as quickly as possible. But is such treatment even necessary?[63]

The demands placed on our physical functioning remain the same for a long period of time. They only change when we age and our body becomes less able to recover. In order to carry out the different functions in the body as effectively as possible, new 'set points' for hormones are established. A higher insulin level means, for example, that you can retain more energy so that you have reserves to use if you need to recover from a potential illness. When you are thirty and your body is still able to recover effectively, it doesn't need that. But once you reach old age, new hormonal set values are established for the first time in a long while.

The production of prolactin, the pituitary hormone that stimulates the mammary glands to produce milk, decreases – after all, it makes no sense for a sixty-year-old woman to produce breast milk. For reasons that are not yet clear, the activity of the thyroid gland also decreases in older people. Initially, doctors suspected that this organ functions less effectively due to old age,[64] but they later established that a less active thyroid gland actually reduces the risk of strokes and heart rhythm disorders. The reference values for blood tests in older people have since been amended. As a result, we don't have to treat every older person with deviating hormone levels – which are the result of a newly configured balance – for illness.

The same also applies to insulin, the hormone that keeps our blood sugar level low. In a fasted state, older people often have a larger amount of glucose in their blood, and higher insulin levels, than younger people.[65] This fits the picture of insulin resistance. But we now know that this is a normal response, so we shouldn't immediately jump to the conclusion that older people have 'age-related diabetes'.

How are the set points for this last phase of life established at the right level? Researchers suspect that the answer lies in the operation of our in-built hormonal feedback system. This is another example of just how clever our endocrine system is. It closely monitors all hormone levels and works like a thermostat, continually adjusting hormone levels depending on what our body needs at that time. Is there too much of a certain hormone? If so, the stimulus that promotes the production of this substance is suppressed. Vice versa: if there is a hormonal shortage, the brake is automatically released so production can be resumed.

In most cases this type of hormonal feedback system ensures that the balance – the homeostasis – is maintained. On the other hand, sometimes the aim is to adjust hormone levels when our body is going through a certain developmental phase. This applies to fertility, for example. In early puberty, the sex organs become more active. So as not to impede this process, the body adjusts the sensitivity of the sex hormone glands with regard to the feedback signal, so the stimulus from the pituitary gland can remain high and the process of becoming fertile can be initiated.[66] Something similar happens as you enter old age, and the pituitary gland plays an important role here too. In the same way that becoming fertile is one of the first new set points in the human body, a decreasing level of sex hormones represents the start of your 'second adolescence', which starts around the age of sixty. For the operation of the pituitary gland, see the diagram on page 49.

Other hormones also start acting differently as you age. The growth hormone variant IGF-1, and the adrenal gland hormone DHEA, similar to testosterone, drop to extremely low levels,[67] while levels of LH and FSH increase – which has additional benefits, as you will see. This can all cause considerable fluctuations to the blood levels, and considering how many different functions each of our hormones have, it is almost as if the body has to learn to walk all over again. In this case, the saying 'once learned, never forgotten' doesn't seem to apply.

An adjusted homeostasis is one of the clearest manifestations of the ageing process. Your body is developing. If the 'healthy norm' *doesn't* change, you and your doctor may see anomalies and symptoms of disease. This may make it difficult to differentiate between certain physiological changes associated with ageing and symptoms of disease. Think of the menopause: what may be a hindrance for one woman may hardly bother someone else. As hormones often have more than one function, our new set points can also present themselves as blessings in disguise.

Take, for example, the rising levels of LH and FSH, which stimulate your sex organs. As the reproductive task is dropped, the continued stimulation of the depleted ovaries and other glands may seem like wasted effort. So scientists wondered whether these hormones controlled by the pituitary gland might fulfil other roles in older age. And they were right; it turns out LH and FSH have several strings to their bow: they're also important for bone density, fat storage, body temperature and an effective memory.[68] Did you know, for example, that Alzheimer's disease is twice as common in women as it is in men? This difference is caused by different LH levels in their blood;a lower LH level in women negatively impacts their memory. [69,70,71,72]

Interfering with these processes isn't necessarily wrong and can even have a positive effect, but only if the complex process has been properly understood and well researched. Supplementing hormones is thus not always the best decision.

## Coming and going

'There's a time for coming and there's a time for going.' These words, written by the Dutch poet and theologian Petrus Augustus de Génestet, also apply to our hormones. They not only have their daily and monthly rhythms, but they also rise and fall during the various phases of life. In older age, sex hormones drop to levels comparable with those before puberty. And although pituitary hormones go into overdrive to compensate for this, they too naturally fall after a few years.

The two lines that follow from de Génestet's poem, 'That's what you heard, but did you understand it too?', are no less applicable. That's precisely the question, if you consider all the desperate (and failed) attempts to rejuvenate ourselves by boosting our hormone levels to those of our younger selves. To date, all efforts to develop a hormonal rejuvenating cure have failed to deliver (and more often than not have led to negative outcomes).

But it's understandable that people continue to experiment in this field; research shows that a decrease in specific hormone levels brings with it so many physical and mental complaints.

Other hormones display a decline similar to sex hormones, but science hasn't yet established a reason for this. As hormones generally fulfil more than one role in the body, Richard Bribiescas – whom I mentioned in the previous chapter – believes that hormones may provide an evolutionary advantage besides their primary role.[74] Many genes in which hormones are involved have remained well preserved for thousands of years – even in animal species without endocrine systems – and this suggests that these hormones fulfil more functions than we may realise. Think, for example, of the role of FSH, which acts as the catalyst of oestrogen production during an earlier stage, but may also be involved in the regulation of body temperature in older women.[75] It's possible that the relatively recent changes to our living conditions, such as greater food security and increasing obesity levels, will mean that these functions will disappear in the distant future.

## Hara hachi bun me

Instead of supplementing hormonal deficits to restore them to the levels experienced during puberty, it would make more sense to ask ourselves how people can age in a healthy way.[76] The simple answer is: by not eating too much and by embracing old age. We can actively influence how we age through our diet simply by only eating until we are 80 per cent full. We can use the population of the prefecture of Okinawa in southern Japan as an example. With their motto *hara hachi bun me* ('eat until you are eight tenths full'), the residents of this region joke that eight of the ten mouthfuls serve the person, and the remaining two the doctor.[77] With their low-calorie but extremely nutritious diet, they are residents of one of the world's 'blue zones': places where life expectancy and health are strikingly higher than average.[78] Besides lower concentrations of insulin, the people of Okinawa have more of the adrenal gland hormone DHEA – similar to testosterone – in their blood.[79] This steroid hormone normally peaks in young adults, after which it drastically decreases, ending up at between 20 and 30 per cent of that value in western adults between the ages of seventy and eighty. This makes it a good marker of someone's biological age. DHEA is also very active in our brain, where it fuels the nerve cells.[80] Researchers investigating the link between DHEA and the health of the residents of Okinawa hoped that this might be a way to boost our health.[81] Extra DHEA does not, however, halt hormonal ageing.[82] Increasing the DHEA concentration in the blood by taking tablets therefore doesn't, in itself, make you any healthier. It seems more likely that the levels of this hormone in these healthy Japanese people are so high because they move a lot and consume fewer calories: both stimulate the release of DHEA. It is therefore more an effect than a cause of healthy ageing.

The fact remains that there's a lot going on in hormonal terms during this phase of life for elderly people in the west. Women become hairier, more wrinkly and more authoritative, whereas men become balder, gentler and somewhat gloomier. Although women and men become more similar as far as hormones are concerned, they remain different in many other regards. The main conclusion is: where lifestyle changes can't help, some supplements can be used to alleviate the worst symptoms that come with old age. But we should exercise caution when considering medication, remembering that our endocrine system is complex and side effects are common.

# 10

# Old Age

*The Beginning of the End*

Once a year, Ludo comes to my surgery. At the age of 94, the widower is still full of life and spends half the year on one of the Spanish costas. Although he shuffles into my surgery with a slightly hunched back, it strikes me that he always seems younger and sprightlier than his age would suggest. He often makes a remark about how he likes to flirt with the ladies and how he hasn't 'lost his touch'. With his sumptuous grey hair, Ludo still looks extremely good and, above all, jovial; I've never once heard him complain. He has a slim, wiry build and, despite an arthritic hip, shoulders and knees, he gets up out of his chair with relative ease.

As he leaves, he cheerfully announces that the array of age-related diseases – an underactive thyroid, prediabetes and high blood pressure – won't get the better of him and that 'the glass is still half full'. Even after his recent cataract operation – 'I can see like an eagle again' – he has managed to continue living independently with just a bit of assistance. He doesn't eat a lot and normally sticks to fish, vegetables and a small glass of wine.

Ludo doesn't feel old ('Doctor, I feel about fifty') and as a retired PE teacher he is used to plenty of exercise; this is something he kept up after retirement. In Spain, he swims in the sea every day and walks along the beach to the neighbouring village to do the shopping. The six-mile round trip, which he would have once been able to run in under an hour, takes him four to five hours. His optimistic outlook and his constitution (which he has managed to maintain his whole life through lots of exercise) make Ludo a healthy old man.

In this final chapter I will describe the role of hormones on mental and physical health during the last phase of life in elderly people. I will also discuss what we can do (sometimes even even decades in advance) to grow old in the healthiest possible way.

What happens, in terms of hormones, from the age of eighty onwards? Three changes take place in the oldest senior citizens: they lose contact with their circadian rhythm as a result of worse sleep quality, which disrupts the production of hormones; the quality of their bones and muscles continues to decrease; and their sense of smell deteriorates. As people aged eighty and above experience loss of appetite and therefore eat less, they are also less fit in general. These factors mutually reinforce each other – a reduced appetite and lower intake of food in turn cause worse sleep and fewer hormones being released.

The first person to refer to the disruption of this hormonal balance in elderly people, before the Second World War, was the American physiologist Walter Cannon.[1] He developed the theory of homeostasis, building on the findings of his French colleague Claude Bernard. Cannon claimed that a person's physiological reserves, which can restore their physical equilibrium, decrease as the person ages. This results in poorer outcomes in the event of illness. This is why I often tell junior doctors that with an elderly patient, once the house of cards starts to wobble, things rarely end well. The limits have been reached.

It's no different for their hormonal balance. As already mentioned, the 24-hour rhythm of our biological clock (also known as the circadian rhythm – *circa* means 'around', *dies* means 'day') is disrupted when our sleeping pattern changes, which also disrupts the release of hormones. The concentrations of hormones during the day have less-pronounced peaks and troughs (a lower pulsatility), similar to low and high tide. The elderly body responds to this by continually producing more hormones such as insulin or leptin, resulting in a type of resistance.[2] It's precisely the fluctuations between high and low concentrations that ensure the body functions properly, enabling it to respond flexibly during periods of illness. The loss of hormonal flexibility, which leads to slightly elevated cortisol levels, is a reliable predictor of dementia and premature death among elderly people.[3,4]

Another important hormonal change is that the sex hormones (notably testosterone) decrease even more at this age, which leads to a dramatic decline in muscle quality.[5] The body also produces less vitamin D and the gut therefore absorbs less calcium, which means the production of parathyroid hormone (PTH) has to increase for sufficient calcium to be released from the bones for adequate blood levels. The result is osteoporosis. Decreasing sex hormones make the optic nerve and the ear work less effectively, causing our sight and hearing to deteriorate.[6,7] The consequences can be disastrous for elderly people; as we are more prone to falls, we're more likely to break bones, which are then less likely to heal properly.

# Eternal life

Although we now know our hormones can do many things, there is one feature in particular that attracts a lot of interest: the opportunity to extend life.[8] In 1939, the English scientist Aldous Huxley (yes, the author of *Brave New World*) wrote *After Many a Summer*,[9] set in California (to where Huxley had just moved at the time), in which he ridicules the temptation to stay forever young. The main character, Jo Stoyte, is a millionaire who is scared to death of dying and therefore wants to live as long as possible. He decides to hire Dr Obispo to see what is scientifically possible. Obispo, inspired by the diaries of the Fifth Earl of Gonister, who had frantically attempted to find the secret to eternal life two hundred years earlier, suggests that the consumption of carp guts and their contents (i.e. a type of faecal transplantation) may have a beneficial effect. At the end of the book, Stoyte and Obispo visit the Fifth Earl of Gonister, who is still alive but now lives in a dungeon and resembles an ape. Jo Stoyte decides not to undergo the treatment after all. What's interesting is that a few years before Huxley finished his novel, he studied carp to find out how they can live for so long (more than a hundred years, he believed).

The British gerontologist and bioinformatician Aubrey de Grey is the oft-quoted apostle of the 'immortality gospel', which is based on growth hormones. His interest in human immortality (and what we can learn about it from other animal species) is certainly nothing new – in fact, this fascination goes back hundreds of years. De Grey believes that, as in the Old Testament, we can live to a thousand as long as we ensure our organs have regular maintenance.[10] This would involve the body's cells being consistently replaced with stem cells. This is what his research has focused on for the past two decades, and one of the substances he puts his proverbial money on is the hormone melatonin.

One of the first accounts of the pursuit of eternal life dates back to around two and a half centuries before Christ. After watching the suffering and death of his best friend Enkidu, Gilgamesh, demigod and king of South Mesopotamia,[11] decided to make the discovery of a rejuvenating elixir his life goal. Out of fear of suffering the same fate as his friend, he visited numerous sages to find out how he could prevent his own demise. One of his advisors was Utnapishtim – literally, 'he who saw life' – the heroic survivor of the oldest flood myth (similar to that of Noah) and himself immortal due to his relationship with the Goddess of Life.[12] Utnapishtim told Gilgamesh that eternal life could be found at the bottom of the ocean.

Gilgamesh's own pursuit failed, but his example has been widely followed. Around thirty years ago, the German biology student Christian Sommer made a chance discovery while researching plankton in seawater off the coast of northern Italy.[13] Miniscule jellyfish were found in the water samples, but once they entered the laboratory these animals appeared to change form. Slowly but surely, they reverted back to their primary state, like butterflies becoming caterpillars again. The animal in question was *Turritopsis dohrnii*: the 'immortal jellyfish'. This is still the only known species of animal that, after successfully developing into an 'adult', can revert back to its original state and subsequently resurrect itself as a healthy creature.[14] This process takes place in response to physical or environmental stress. One of the internal triggers for the reverse life cycle of the jellyfish is reaching a certain age: old age. Three guesses for which actors hold sway here: hormones! Believe it or not, the rejuvenating hormones that regulate this process in jellyfish appear to be controlled by substances akin to our growth hormone.[15]

## Everyone as old as Father Christmas?

Over the past fifty years, life expectancy in the Netherlands has increased by around 13 per cent, or almost ten years.[16] The life expectancy for a baby born in 1970 was 70.9 for a boy and 76.5 for a girl, but by 2021 this had increased to 79.7 for men and 83 for women. In future, it is looking less likely that we will be able to speak of a population pyramid. More and more people are living longer, and not only in the Netherlands. It's estimated that by 2050, there will be just as many over sixty-fives in the world as fifteen-year-olds. This is mainly thanks to the improved living conditions that are reducing the risk of death in our younger years. It doesn't mean that people didn't get old in the past, but the chance of getting old was smaller.[17] With a record of one hundred and twenty two years of age, Homo sapiens are still a way off the awe-inspiring age of Methuselah, who is said in the Bible to have lived to nine hundred and sixty nine years old. Humans don't fare well in life expectancy compared to related animals, like apes, which can live up to four times longer. While we have to make do with made-up stories about growing younger – like the film *The Curious Case of Benjamin Button* or Virginia Woolf's novel *Orlando*, the life story of a young poet who changes from a man into a woman throughout his three-hundred-year life – this is the order of the day for the immortal jellyfish.

Research shows that humans can, however, add years to their life, and this understanding has consequences for our attitudes towards old age and death. Although most scientists and inhabitants of the earth see our demise as an unavoidable part of life,[18] others (led by Aubrey de Grey) believe it must also be possible for humans to push back manifestations of ageing and thereby prolong life. In future, old age could fall under the list of 'conditions' we can treat. This different way of thinking has inspired researchers to seek the limits of our physiological possibilities in the way an elite athlete works towards a new personal best. With a growing population of older people, it's important for the sustainability of a society that its oldest members become *healthier*. Health will enable them to live longer without relying on the support of the younger generations.

The opportunity to live for centuries, like Enoch and Methuselah in the Old Testament, is not yet within arm's reach, but a better understanding of our hormones (among other things) could change this. In the previous chapter we saw that simple hormone supplementation isn't the solution. But the more studies that are carried out and hypotheses tested, the more we're seeing results gradually improving. Scientists are gaining a better understanding of what happens, on a hormonal level, as we age. It seems that in this phase a reorganisation takes place in the hormonal head office. And the chief conductor of all of this is hidden deep within the brain.

## The hypothalamus as the clock of life

As far back as 1929, the American neurosurgeon Harvey Cushing said that the hypothalamus is where the source of our life is located.[19] It's fitting, therefore, that it's located close to the pineal gland, which Descartes said was the seat of the soul.[20] In the previous chapters, we have already encountered the hypothalamus a few times. It's as small as a thumbnail but extremely influential. It acts like a type of traffic controller to ensure good hormonal health. It controls our behaviour for survival: it makes sure (via hunger, thirst and satiety stimuli) that we eat and drink enough so that we have enough energy for a 'fight or flight' response in the event of danger (preparing your body for action) and that we have sex in order to reproduce. The hypothalamus also controls our biological clock (circadian rhythm) and body temperature.

What's striking is that the bodily functions that the hypothalamus controls often get disrupted in old age. This led scientists to wonder whether, in addition to the circadian rhythm, the hypothalamus also controls the timing of the phases of life, like a treasure chest full of life energy. It seemed that Cushing was right, because now, a good century after his hunch, researchers are presenting proof that the hypothalamus plays a prominent role in the initiation of the ageing process throughout the body.

The 'jewels' in the treasure chest (the 'source', according to Cushing) could well be our stem cells: special undifferentiated cells that can develop into almost any type of cell from which our body is made: skin, blood, muscle, brain. It's been known for a long time that bone marrow contains stem cells, but research has now revealed that the hypothalamus also has a supply of them. These stem cells in the hypothalamus, at least in mice, appear to be the key to the cause of ageing, as stem cells are no longer found in the hypothalamus of two-year-old mice (the equivalent to a seventy- to eighty-year-old person). An additional dose can extend life expectancy by the equivalent of a good eleven human years.[21]

This is all to do with cell division. The cells in our body are renewed in an assembly line; a type of continuous maintenance activity whereby worn components are replaced. This is how the body keeps tissues healthy. Old, damaged cells are cleared away by the immune system, and healthy cells then divide to restore the cell's power. The cells in some organs have to be replaced more quickly than others, but generally this process means that

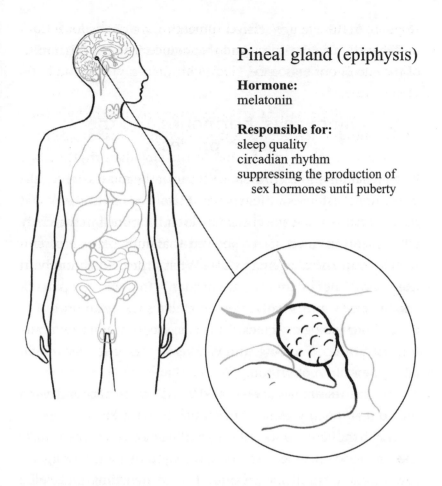

## Pineal gland (epiphysis)

**Hormone:**
melatonin

**Responsible for:**
sleep quality
circadian rhythm
suppressing the production of
    sex hormones until puberty

every seven to ten years, a large part of a person's body (including all of their fat tissue) is replaced.[22]

If you are young your cells are continually renewed, and this process becomes increasingly important as you age. Stem cells are found in organs throughout the entire body, including the skin, brain, liver, blood and, above all, bone marrow. They're responsible for the renewal impulse and can, for example, cause a large part of a liver to regenerate. The supply may appear endless – a stem cell can also generate new stem cells – but it isn't. That's because even though the constant renewal of stem cells would be handy for age-related ailments, the maintenance team of stem cells also declines. And that could mean the beginning of the end of our existence.

## Stem cells, hormones and the ageing process

As you age, the supply of stem cells decreases and the stem cells in the hypothalamus suffer the same fate. You might think that the lower the supply, the closer to the end you are, but the study with mice described above showed that supplementing stem cells keeps physical ageing at bay. What's the connection with hormones? These stem cells are primarily found in the parts of the hypothalamus involved in producing the hormones that control our biological clock. This suggests that hormonal factors may influence ageing, and vice versa: ageing sets hormonal adjustments in motion too.

The same researchers investigated this theory in mice and determined that the tiny gland communicates the start of the ageing process to the body via so-called signalling molecules. These make the 'life clock' influence the biological rhythms of certain organs. We're already familiar with one of these signalling molecules: GnRH, produced by the hypothalamus itself (see Chapter 1). The main function of this hormone is to stimulate your sex organs to produce sex hormones. A decreasing supply of stem cells corresponds with a lower production of GnRH, as this hormone dips as you age.[23] Mice with elevated GnRH levels not only lost fewer brain cells and performed better cognitively, they also remained young in other regards, such as muscle strength, bone mass and connective tissue. The rejuvenating strategy in these mice also led to an increase in sex hormones, which could explain why we age more rapidly as soon as our fertility comes to an end.

GnRH is not the only signalling molecule produced by the hypothalamus. The stem cells themselves also produce signalling proteins that keep everything in balance; a smaller quantity of stem cells also results in fewer signalling proteins, causing your whole body to age.[24] This can lead to the above-mentioned changes to the daily hormone levels.

## Your biological age: healthy ageing

When we talk about age, we automatically think of someone's calendar age: the time that has passed since they were born. But this number doesn't always correspond with the *biological* age, which describes whether someone is ageing in a healthy way. Two people over the age of eighty could have a similar calendar age but differ drastically in terms of fitness (and therefore life expectancy).[25] Using the slogan '*Je echte leeftijd*' ('Your real age'), TV advertisements, programmes and books familiarised the Dutch public with this concept a few years ago. People were invited to fill in a questionnaire on special websites to calculate the difference between their calendar age and biological age.[26] Information about lifestyle (exercise, diet, smoking and drinking habits), stress and body weight was then used to produce a positive result – a lower biological age than calendar age – or a negative one. Participants were then provided with advice depending on the results. Although these factors can give an impression of health *behaviour*, this kind of questionnaire can't precisely determine a person's physical fitness.

So how should we establish someone's biological age? We currently use measurable data like eye lens thickness and grip strength, which are a good reflection of someone's biological age.[27] The search for objective biological markers (biomarkers) that can be used to assess fitness is, however, not a straightforward one. Since the 1960s, scientists have been looking for pieces of the puzzle to use to determine a person's biological age. As part of this they've investigated hormones like DHEA, which cropped up in the previous chapter in connection with the senior citizens of Okinawa in Japan, who remain remarkably fit as they age.[28] This adrenal gland hormone, known as the 'mother of all hormones' because it can be converted into sex hormones in the body, has been the subject of great interest because researchers believed that higher concentrations in the blood could be associated with better health in older age. As we saw earlier, however, treatments using this hormone didn't have favourable results.[29,30]

## Searching for the land of Nod

In Chapter 3 I outlined the importance of sleep, diet and exercise in the hormonal health of adolescents. It's not entirely coincidental that these factors also apply to the elderly in the last phase of life. In the hormonal traffic, rush hour takes place at night. During the deep, slow-wavelength sleep in particular, lots of growth hormone is released into the blood. Like adolescents, elderly people lack the good quality of sleep necessary for the regeneration and development of muscle and bone tissue. Their sleep is less efficient (shorter and more superficial) with fewer deep, slow-wave sleep phases.[31] In older people, the neural pathway between the retina and the hypothalamus (the retino-hypothalamic tract, which controls the release of melatonin in the pineal gland) functions less effectively, impacting the production and release of the sleep hormone melatonin.[32,33] Incidentally, the same thing happens with blind people, who appear to be afflicted by a disrupted circadian rhythm throughout their lives because the neural pathway no longer functions.[34]

A large-scale Dutch sleep study carried out by Eus van Someren, a professor of neurophysiology at VU Amsterdam, revealed that older people are especially prone to insomnia: the inability to fall asleep.[35] But if you want to make it to a hundred, research shows just how important it is to get at least eight hours' sleep a night – an afternoon nap is certainly not the solution.[36] Most elderly people don't have such a favourable sleep pattern and, as with adolescents, a disrupted circadian rhythm directly affects the production of growth and stress hormones, which are already compromised. This ultimately results in elevated cholesterol and blood sugar levels, which diminishes the body's ability to repair itself.

There is hope on the horizon, however, for elderly people who sleep badly: daily melatonin taken in the form of low-dosage tablets appears to have some effect.[37] A healthy lifestyle is still much more effective than medication, though: don't sit around too much, and get plenty of exercise outdoors and in the sunshine. Movement increases the production of melatonin and improves sleep quality.[38] You're also advised to avoid blue light from your phone the hour before you go to sleep and to move heavier meals to the afternoon.[39,40] In other words, you can help yourself find the way to the land of Nod by embracing a healthy lifestyle.

## Physical activity

Physical activity naturally stimulates the production and release of sleep hormones like melatonin,[41] but has an even bigger effect on growth hormones. As you age, the levels of muscle-building (anabolic) hormones like testosterone and growth hormone decrease, yet physical activity can boost hormonal levels in the elderly. More muscle mass means less chance of falling and a more effective metabolism (as was the case with my patient Ludo). On average, an eighty-year-old man has already lost around half of the muscle mass he has built up over his life-time.[42,43] The greater the loss of muscle mass, the greater the chance of age-related disease and death.[44] That's why it becomes increasingly important to regularly do both endurance and strength training as you age.

A case like Ludo's shows that sometimes calendar age says nothing about someone's biological age.[45] The same applies to the elderly people in the documentary *Autumn Gold* who train daily for the World Masters Athletics Championships.[46] Despite the lower basic levels of testosterone and growth hormone with age, research shows that regular exercise increases growth hormone in men over the age of eighty. The effect of exercise has been less well-researched in women, but we can safely say that thirty minutes of physical activity a day is an effective way to counteract the loss of muscle and bone quality in older women too (supplemented with half an hour of brain exercise like solving a crossword puzzle).[47]

## About people and their smell

The only thing Ludo complains about is that people tell him he doesn't smell particularly pleasant after exercising. 'Can you not do something about that, doctor?'

Smell gives us an indication of how healthy or ill a body is: our nose can make us aware of this. We certainly know someone who always smells of musk, while someone else often seems to be surrounded by an odour of rancid butter. But we also use our nose in the medical field on an almost daily basis. Every doctor knows the strong smell in the breath of a liver patient in the final stage of their disease. And they're also familiar with the pungent odour that accompanies the start of a urinary tract infection or the sweet-smelling urine that doctors once used to establish the hormonal disease diabetes mellitus (without having a cure for it). I use my nose mainly in the foot wound clinic when I try to guess, on the basis of a sickly-sweet smell, which bacterial infection corresponds with a wound (of course a bacterial culture provides the definitive answer a few days later).

We're fascinated with smells in our daily lives too. As far back as 200 BC, Aristotle tried to determine why our armpits sweat.[48] His answer: because there is hardly any ventilation and cooling there. And why doesn't our body smell when we eat something smelly? According to the Greek philosopher, as soon as you eat something that smells bad, its smell is replaced by your own smell!

Besides emitting odours via pheromones, we also emit them through our faeces, breath, urine, blood, saliva, vaginal fluids and, of course, our skin. In the skin, we have two types of glands that secrete fluids: exocrine glands secrete the watery sweat solution from the skin, and apocrine glands in the hair follicles secrete sebum, an oily substance that protects your skin from drying out. It's usually the latter, in combination with skin bacteria and UV light, that give us a bad smell. While freshly produced skin oils (lipids) may still smell like sweet lemon, after contact with air and sunlight this pleasant smell changes to a cutting, musk-like odour. The amount of sebum secretion also differs between people of European and African origin and those of Asian origin. The apocrine sweat glands of African and European people produce a sticky type of sebum that results in a cheesy body odour, whereas Asian people don't have this so-called ABCC11 transporter and therefore produce a dry, crumbly sebum.[49] Our sex hormones also influence our sebum production.[50]

Our diet and our gut microbiome (see Chapter 6) determine what our faeces smell like. They can be sickly sweet or sour, if we've eaten lots of dairy products, and can smell like ammonia or sulphur if we have eaten lots of protein or cabbage. The question is whether food also influences the way our skin smells. The substances that are removed remain behind in our faeces, but also travel throughout our whole body and can produce pleasant or unpleasant smells there too. Research confirms this. In one study, the smell of breast-fed babies had a pleasant effect on mothers who had just given birth as well as those who had never had children. Brain scans clearly showed that the dopaminergic reward system in the adults was activated.[51] Other research has shown that mothers with more cortisol (stress hormone) in their saliva – those who are therefore more 'switched on' – are better able to recognise the smell of their own baby and become calmer as a result.[52] Speaking from experience, this also applies to men. When my son was in his hospital bed for months on end for his cancer treatment, I often sought comfort at home by sniffing his pyjamas, to shake off those feelings of stress.

TMAO (trimethylamine N-oxide) is one of the best-known odours from our faeces and can give us an indication of our health as adults. It smells like rotten fish and is released by proteins in our gut microbiome.[53] The smell is an important indicator of cardiovascular disease and kidney damage. Faecal transplantation studies have shown that cresols (which smell likes a horse's stable) can also be an indicator of these conditions, and that we ought to be aware if there's a lower presence of butyric acid and acetic acid in our blood.[54,55] This is because butyric acid and acetic acid have a beneficial effect on our food intake, energy balance and the immune system.[56] We're all familiar with the bad breath you get after a night out; this says a lot about your body's metabolism at that moment. Medical technology is currently being developed based on a type of electronic 'nose' that picks up certain smells in exhaled air for the early detection of cancer, gastrointestinal disorders and lung disease.[57]

Let's now return to Ludo and his concerns about his body odour. It is true that older people have a different body odour to younger people.[58] Older Americans apparently smell like aromatic beeswax, whereas older Japanese people smell like cucumber.[59] In both cases, younger people find the smell of old people less pleasant than their own smell, which is like butter.[60] The Japanese refer to the body odour of older people as *kareishu*, which means something akin to 'old man's smell', as Harold McGee describes in his book *Nose Dive*.[61]

I can hear you saying: *Haven't I already read something about that?* And yes, these substances could very well be pheromones, which give us an indication of the age and intentions of a person before we have even spoken to them. This enables us to estimate someone's age relatively reliably based on their body odour. And like pheromones, some body odours (produced by skin bacteria) send signals to our hypothalamus to control our production of hormones.[62,63]

None of this solves Ludo's problem, but it does explain why he doesn't smell great to the outside world. One positive, however, is that our sense of smell continuously declines as we age, so the older person themselves is less and less bothered by it.[64]

# Digestion and appetite: compliments to the hormones

The effects of hormonal changes are also reflected in the eating habits of older people. Many people over the age of eighty start eating differently due to their age, but also to reduced fitness levels. While adolescents can stuff their faces and rarely feel full as they approach adulthood, older bodies generally release fewer hunger cues.[65] Their appetite decreases and they snack less often too.[66] Older people also crave certain foods less,[67] which is probably related to changed levels of digestive hormones such as cholecystokinin (CCK) and the satiety hormone leptin.[68,69] This, in combination with slightly altered ghrelin levels,[70] means that older people become less interested in food.

The finding that digestive processes work differently in older people is a recent but important one because malnutrition is prevalent in this group. Another age-related ailment that contributes to this eating pattern is a dry mouth and a distorted sense of taste. In all cases, these processes are the result of hormonal changes.[71]

The complex process of digestion starts in the mouth, where food products are literally 'prepared' by the saliva. In Chapter 3, we discovered that saliva contains important hormones that enable you to taste whether someone could be the right partner for you. At an older age, you produce less saliva, which makes chewing and swallowing more difficult.[72] Your taste itself is also controlled by hormones via receptors on the tongue – this is how leptin, for example, reduces cravings for sweet things.[73]

The combination of a dry mouth and an altered sense of taste due to changed digestive hormones therefore directly influences the quantity and quality of our food intake and our appetite. One of the best-known examples of this is the 'changed sense of taste' during pregnancy, when the expectant mother suddenly no longer enjoys her favourite foods (see Chapter 1). In older people too, a disrupted sense of taste is probably also an evolutionary adaptation mechanism that makes mammals instinctively choose food and drink containing nutrients suited to a specific life phase. So it may not be entirely surprising that young children aren't so keen on grandma's salty stews, whereas more salt for grandma increases her blood pressure, decreasing her risk of falling or fainting.[74]

Older people who (partially) lose their sense of taste can end up either underweight or overweight. If you eat less or a very limited range of foods because you can no longer taste certain flavours well, you're at risk of losing weight. This applies especially to people over the age of eighty, who already have fewer reserves due to their age and are at greater risk of illness in the event of weight loss.[75] Of course, the question that then arises is whether here, too, the hypothalamus can be the catalyst for maintaining a healthy weight in older people. This makes this hormonal head office an interesting target for anti-ageing strategies.

The hypothalamus appears to be involved in both the release of hormones by endocrine glands and the quality of bone and muscle mass, and the perception of taste and hunger.[76] For that reason, scientists from all over the world believe it must be possible to reset the personal life clock of various organs via the hypothalamus, and even attempt to turn back the biological clock by transferring blood from young animals to old ones.[77] Apparently the blood of young animals contains substances that counteract ageing. Unfortunately we don't know yet which substances these are in humans. In the pursuit of an elixir of life, blood transfusions are therefore not seen as a real option. So much for the modern Dracula myth!

## The big clean-up

Why wouldn't anyone who can afford it want to invest money into research regarding eternal youth? For the Amazon billionaire Jeff Bezos, it has never been in question. He invested millions of dollars in a start-up company called Unity Biotechnology, which develops medicines designed to counter ageing.[78] This decision has likely either financially motivated or a result of his eternal competition with the founders of Google, who established Calico – a company with the same objective – in 2013.[79] But in view of Bezos's recent escapades in space, it may well be the case that he wants to contribute to his own immortality.[80] If we want to turn back our universal biological clock, like the immortal jellyfish, it seems sensible not only to boost our hormone levels, but also to counteract the natural demise of stem cells.

One of the physical processes that causes the supply of stem cells to rapidly decrease is the formation of so-called zombie cells. Here, we need to return to cell division, which cannot continue indefinitely. There is a limit to the number of cell divisions that can take place before our DNA is damaged. The chromosomes of our DNA have protective ends – telomeres – that become slightly shorter with each division. From the moment that these telomeres become too short to permit another cell division without important DNA information being lost, a cell finds itself in a type of zombie mode: division is no longer possible, but 'self-destruction' is not an option either.[81]

These zombie cells are our old-age cells. They're found throughout our entire body and appear in all tissues sooner or later. They make our skin wrinkle and our organs less fit. And however inactive the word 'zombie' may sound, these cells unfortunately remain very active in one field: inflammation. The more these cells accumulate, the more readily our body responds with a chronic inflammatory reaction, including in the hypothalamus.[82] Stem cells are very sensitive to this inflammatory environment, causing them to rapidly decrease in number. Recovery of the organ becomes impossible and we noticeably decline.

Experiments into the field of extending human life are being carried out using medicines that selectively clean up the zombie cells. This is a bit like a big spring clean. These experimental drugs are called senolytics, which literally means 'dismantling of ageing'. One of the pioneers in this field is the Dutch cell biologist Jan van Deursen, who, together with his American research team, gave a senolytic drug to mice for the first time in 2011.[83] This drug relieved the animals of their old-age cells and the associated ailments by reducing the number of zombie cells by around 30 per cent. As a nice side effect, the bone quality and hormonal balance of these lucky mice also increased. The treatment is based on a previous experiment that had the same cleaning-up effect in fat cells.[84] It emerged that there's one specific messenger that influences our metabolism as well as our life expectancy: human growth hormone. We already know from the events in puberty that our growth hormone is crucial to our metabolism and the storage of fat. But the hormone is also increasingly being associated with a longer, and above all healthier, life expectancy.

These results made Aubrey de Grey wonder whether hormonal interventions held the key to eternal life.[85] But some individuals – like the American real estate millionaire Darren Moore – don't want to sit around waiting for the results of the companies associated with Amazon and Google, so have instead decided to offer themselves up as human guinea pigs. Moore is injecting himself with FOX01, the substance that may be responsible for immortality in the eponymous jellyfish, and he takes senolytic drugs on a daily basis.[86] He hopes that the ageing process will grind to a halt or, better still, that his biological age will decrease.

It's worth stressing that scientists like Van Deursen warn us not to look at the current situation through rose-tinted glasses.[87] Senolytics may seem promising when it comes to keeping our hormone levels in check, but so far they have mainly been tested on mice; they've not yet been proven to be effective in humans too. Prematurely giving people senolytics could lead to health problems.

As yet there's no hormonal miracle pill to prevent our dreaded cellular decline, but as long as there's life there's hope. And under the motto 'prevention is better than cure', there may be another way of using hormones to counteract ageing.

# The first immortal woman

Henrietta Lacks was born in the US state of Virginia in 1920, where she spent her life as a tobacco worker. At the age of thirty-one she went to the Johns Hopkins Hospital in Baltimore complaining of severe stomach pain. There she was diagnosed with metastatic cervical cancer, from which she died a short while later. But Henrietta Lacks is technically still alive today, and not only in the book by Rebecca Skloot.[88]

Without Lacks realising it, her doctors removed tumour cells during her stay in the hospital for the purpose of research into possible treatments – something that would not be permitted under today's regulations on medical ethics. Human material often has a limited life, but Henrietta's cells, now better known as HeLa cells, survived for an exceptionally long time. In fact, they simply wouldn't die. The miraculous immortality of her cells enabled medical research to be carried out on a huge scale. I was involved with such research myself in the laboratory in San Diego; the cells really grow like crazy! Research into these cells has led to significant breakthroughs in medicine, including an effective vaccine for polio and knowledge about diseases like AIDS and some types of cancer. Tens of thousands of patents have since been linked to the cells, of which there are now so many that their weight is greater than a good hundred Empire State Buildings put together. Unsurprisingly, Henrietta's family started a court case against the company that earned millions from the HeLa cells as well as the hospitals that use the cells in their labs for research.[89]

The reason why the HeLa cells were immortal remained a mystery for a long time, until a trio of scientists discovered the enzyme telomerase in 1984. This discovery, for which Elizabeth Blackburn, Carol Greider and Jack Szostak received the Nobel Prize for Physiology or Medicine in 2009,[90] proved vitally important. Telomerase is a protein found naturally in our stem cells and ensures the extension of a person's telomeres, thereby preventing zombie mode and enabling the cell to survive for longer. If the protein remains active, as was the case with Henrietta, the cell can even survive indefinitely. In her case, there was a mutation in the genetic code which also stimulated the non-stem cells to start making telomerase. This led to uncontrolled growth of tissue and the formation of tumours and cancer. Henrietta died of this disease, but at the same time this genetic deviation gave her cells eternal life.

This makes telomerase extremely interesting when it comes to the pursuit of a longer life.[91] Our telomeres become shorter as we age and shortened telomeres are associated with the start of age-related diseases like cardiovascular disease, cancer and diabetes as well as reduced muscle strength.[92] If we can find a way to control the activity of telomerase – for example, by turning its production on and off – we may be able to rejuvenate our cells. Compliments to the miracle substance that manages that, I hear you say. The good news is that these substances have already been discovered: hormones. While cortisol and chronic stress make the telomeres shrink,[93] a higher level of growth hormone in the blood causes an increased length of the telomere.[94] Exercise and sleep therefore help indirectly too. And then there's the effect of nutrition.

## Quid pro quo

Consume grapes and the red wine derived from them, green tea, and hard-to-pronounce food supplements which can absorb oxygen free radicals in our bodies: this is some of the recent nutritional advice for a longer, healthier life. A number of years ago, the book *The Food Hourglass* by the Belgian doctor and researcher Kris Verburgh drew attention to the influence of our eating habits on the ageing process.[95] In it, Verburgh calls for a new scientific discipline: nutrigerontology, which is a cross between geriatrics and nutrition. He is not the first doctor to recognise the importance of a healthy diet on long-term health, but he is one of the first to partially blame our sugar metabolism for the fact we aren't living as long.

According to him, the chief culprits here are the high-calorie sugars like fructose, which are prevalent in our diet and age our bodies. Scientific proof of this is not always clear,[96] but recent research shows that the hormonal mechanisms activated to digest sugars not only shorten our life expectancy but also increase the number of years we spend in worse health. In laboratory animals, for example, fructose is well-known to impede a longer life.[97] In people too, a diet containing less fructose appears to be important for a healthy old age,[98] as fructose shortens our telomeres.[99] This highly calorific sugar appears, in turn, to directly affect the hormone-regulating functions in laboratory animals via the substance FOX01.[100] Poor nutrition and a lack of exercise reduces this protein in the organs, whereas good nutrition and more exercise increases it.[101,102] This is exactly the same FOX01 mechanism the jellyfish uses to activate its immortality trick.[103]

Living up to eleven years longer because healthy (sugar-free) nutrition leads to more growth hormone and a well-adjusted hypothalamus; a 40 per cent increase in life expectancy by taking certain anti-ageing pills (senolytics): these are significant figures. But if you think that's an impressive example of hormonal power, there's news: it gets even better!

Just before the turn of the century, *Nature* published the findings of American researchers who had discovered that a worm that hadn't reproduced lived longer than its conspecifics who already had offspring.[104] This mechanism again took place via the growth hormone axis. And the same also appears to apply to humans – although mainly to mothers,[105] probably due to all the energy expended and the physical toll a pregnancy can take on a mother's body.[106] Fathers, on the other hand, reach an older age after having daughters (strikingly, having sons doesn't make a difference). The reason for this is unknown, but it's possible that a stereotypical upbringing and the division of roles between men and women, and associated chronic stress levels, play a part.[107] There aren't many young people who would exchange their potential offspring for a longer life. For most people, that's too high a price to pay. Nevertheless, the most reliable way to increase your life expectancy is by not bearing children and avoiding sugar.[108] Studies show that worms with this lifestyle lived up to six times as long, for up to 124 days as opposed to twenty. With this experiment too, researchers are cautiously optimistic about discovering similar mechanisms in people.

# What can you do yourself?

The only question left is: beyond all the promises of medical advances for the future, what can we actually do to age in a healthy way? The answer is easier than you might think: how old you feel says something about how healthy you feel.[109] While this may be difficult to measure in the consulting room, older people who have a positive attitude and/or are people of faith, are often healthier and actually live a number of years longer.[110,111]

Research shows that positive people over the age of eighty-five live a good 10 to 15 per cent longer than their more negatively inclined peers. Gloominess and a poor memory in old age are associated with low concentrations of male and female sex hormones.[112,113] But (as you will have already guessed) treatment using sex hormones doesn't suddenly make gloominess and depression disappear.[114,115]

If pills aren't the solution, what can you do? Write down what you're happy about and grateful for each day and repeat this out loud several times (positive affirmation), spend time exclusively with positive people and have a goal in life (varying from spiritual experiences to living with and for the grandchildren). This will stand you in good stead. A study has shown that mindfulness could also help slow down the ageing process.[116] In short, there aren't yet any pills that extend our life, but there is increasing hope for the modern and positively minded Gilgamesh.

## Old Age

So here are your doctor's orders to maintain your hormonal balance as early as possible in life by eating healthily and getting enough exercise. You should also keep your circadian rhythm on track. There is certainly some truth to the old Dutch saying, 'What you learn in youth, you learn for life.'

# Epilogue

I hope I've been able to convey my fascination with our endocrine system through this book. Over the past century, a great many mysteries have been unravelled about the interaction between hormones and society, as demonstrated in the story of the female pope Joan. Research into endocrine glands and the treatment of endocrine disorders is still far from complete, however, and that is frustrating for a doctor.

It might seem like we can easily detect and treat endocrine disorders, but we're still in the dark about a lot of things. We can't accurately chart the release of hormones from a gland in healthy people, let alone in a *sick* endocrine gland in the event of deviations. As practitioners and patients, we have to make do with a blood test to judge the status of an endocrine gland, and this is only ever a snapshot. If we then start treatment, the process is not all that different to how it would have been half a century ago. Since we can manufacture hormones synthetically, we give our patients medications that they have to take or inject on a daily basis. And although these treatments often result in balanced hormone levels, we can't replicate the ingenious way in which a gland in our body releases hormones.[1] Basically, it's still a rather crude form of treatment and that's probably also the reason why so many patients still have complaints.

I have high expectations of the treatments for diabetes patients, whereby insulin and glucagon are injected into the body by means of a small pump. The most recent version of these insulin pumps has a sensor that can directly measure the effect on blood glucose levels. As the sensor has a self-learning algorithm, this type of insulin pump increasingly becomes part of the patient's body and better imitates the function of a pancreas. In this way, this piece of equipment can predict how much insulin the body needs to keep the blood sugar level as normal as possible.[2] Of course, this is much better than having to inject yourself with insulin four times a day. How great would it be if there was also smart equipment like this for people with an underactive thyroid gland or a defective adrenal gland, or for the production of growth hormone? Fortunately, a recent paper showed that there is a possibility of measuring daily fluctuations in adrenal gland hormones over time with a sensor.[3] This is a promising first step.

However, in my opinion, there's still a lot to be done in the coming decade. It's still difficult to establish how endocrine disorders actually come about and what the connection is between genetic factors, the environment and gut bacteria – let alone having a reliable test that can identify exactly who in our society is at risk of developing a certain disease. We want to be able to offer these people a treatment that can slow down the progression of their disease or, better still, combat it. Only time will tell whether that succeeds – it will, in any case, be very exciting.

Writing this book has been a process of blood, sweat and tears. I underestimated how long it would take to get my thoughts down on paper. This was especially difficult because, as scientists, we are trained to report our research findings in a concise way, but I had to do the opposite here and learn how to get my message across as a narrative. It was an informative process, especially because I kept arriving at the sobering conclusion that we actually know so little about the cause of our diseases.

We live in harmony with the world around us. It's fascinating to see that people in ancient times already knew this and felt inspired to find new treatment methods to alleviate the suffering experienced by their peers. In the oath that doctors take, they have to say: 'I shall promote the medical knowledge of myself and others.'[4] I hope this book has contributed to that.

# Acknowledgements

My father and Diederik van Geel, GPs in Brunssum where I grew up: in your own way, you were both examples of how I work as a doctor today.

Dear Dad, as a GP you were a real people's doctor. As a young boy, you let me join you on home visits to old farms, where residents sometimes only spoke in the Limburg dialect or German. I saw how you made diagnoses and treated patients with ease, and without any equipment.

Diederik, as Roderik's father, you taught me to look at things independently and sometimes more rationally, and how great it can be to play with words and language. It is a shame you are no longer here to witness the publication of this book.

Dear Mum, thank you for sharing all your experiences from the field of nursing in the late 1960s, which you told with great relish at the dining table (how you taught arrogant trainee doctors and assistant doctors a lesson!). Your stories taught me that I should always treat people with love and respect, but that I can also remind them of their responsibilities.

Dear sisters Ilse and Sabine, and your partners Gijsjan and Joeri: thank you for your warmth and support.

Besides a medical degree, Utrecht gave me three things:

friendships for life, the love of my life and my in-laws, the Speelmans, who helped me extend my knowledge about the Bible.

Mrs Nolet, my Greek and Latin teacher: you said in middle school that I'd be better off pursuing the arts than the sciences. I ended up taking a scientific route, but I hope that with this book I have gained my credits for the linguistic side of my education.

Dear Paul Bouter, twenty-two years ago, in the city of Den Bosch, I sat down on a stool beside you as a trainee doctor and assisted you in one of your consulting hours. There, my fascination with endocrinology and diabetes was born.

Dear Marije and Huib de Goeij, in 2011 we spent many months together in the paediatric oncology department at Amsterdam UMC for the treatment of Matthias and Faas. We shared highs and lows. Willemijn and I are grateful to you for the valuable friendship that ensued.

Finally – in no particular order – I would like to thank the following people: Hans Sauerwein, Manon Schreuder, Joost Hoekstra, Paul Lips, Tessa Busch-Westbroek, Martin den Heijer, Mieke Godfried, Frits Holleman, Hans de Vries, Daniël van Raalte, Mark Kramer, Marleen Kemper, Carla Hollak, Michaela Diamant, Robert Heine, Paul van Trotsenburg, Gabor Linthorst, Peter Bisschop, Bart Roep and Mireille Serlie: my educators in endocrinology.

Fredrik Bäckhed, Martin Blaser and Willem de Vos: my educators in the gut microbiome. Erik Stroes, Harry Büller, John Kastelein, Peter Speelman, Marcel Levi, Joost Hoekstra, Jeff Esko: my scientific educators.

Roderik van Geel, Sander Schouten, Rogier van Tooren, Jeroen van Eendenburg, Victor Gerdes, Bert Groen, Pieter Speelman, Jan-Jaap Bakker, Peter Balk, Johan Esselink, Boaz Klein Haneveld,

# Acknowledgements

Celeste Snoek, Friso Verschoor, Mirjam Abdulrahman, Michiel and Marit van de Sande, Pascalle Rademaekers, and Suthesh Sivapalaratnam: thank you for the interesting discussions and valuable friendships.

The members of my student association in Utrecht and the Tastevin in Amsterdam, because they made sure I wasn't just a bookworm and didn't become a workaholic.

Hans Romijn, Eric Fliers, Maarten Soeters and Frida van den Maagdenberg for critically reading the manuscript. Alex Bakker for his feedback on Chapter 4.

Myrthe Frissen: thanks for all of your help with the source research.

Anne Kramer: this book wouldn't be here without you. Haye Koningsveld, Mariska Kortie and Jacqueline de Jong from De Bezige Bij publishers, as well as Catharina Schilder.

Arnold van de Laar, Jet Hopster, Lara Bressser: thank you for your help with the writing process.

My patients and PhD students for all the inspiration.

Willemijn and my children. Life is a blast with you. The glass is and always will be half full!

# Notes

## Foreword

1 Mantel, H. (2003). *Giving Up the Ghost*. London: Fourth Estate.

## Introduction

1 https://www.trouw.nl/nieuws/
professor-galjaard-neemt-afscheid~b513d97e/
2 Bayliss, W.M. & E.H. Starling (1902). 'On the causation of the
so-called "Peripheral Reflex Secretion" of the pancreas'. In: *Proc
Roy Soc*, 69: 352–3.
3 Bayliss, W.M. & E.H. Starling (1902). 'The mechanism of
pancreatic secretion'. In: *J Physiol*, 28: 325–53.
4 https://www.nobelprize.org/prizes/medicine/1904/summary/
5 Berthold, A.A. (1849). 'Transplantation der Hoden'. In: *Archiv
für Anatomie, Physiologie und Wissenschafliche Medicin*. Berlin: J.
Müller, Veit & Co.
6 https://en.wikipedia.org/wiki/Heart_of_a_Dog
7 Cussons, A.J., Bhagat, C.I., Fletcher, S.J. & J.P. Walsh (2002).
'Brown-Séquard Revisited: A Lesson from History on The Placebo
Effect of Androgen Treatment'. In: *J Aust*, Dec 2–16; 177
(11–12): 678–9.
8 Knegtmans, P.J. (2014). *Geld, ijdelheid en hormonen. Ernst Lacqueur
(1880–1947), hoogleraar en ondernemer*. Amsterdam: Boom.
9 Carson, R. (1962). *Silent Spring*. Boston: Houghton Mifflin.
10 Rikken, B. et al. (1996). 'Hypofysair groeihormoon en de ziekte
van Creutzfeldt-Jakob in Nederland'. In: *Ned Tijdschr Geneeskd*,
140: 1163–5.
11 https://www.descentrum.nl/voor-des-dochters

## Chapter 1 – First the Egg, Then the Chicken

1 Stockley, P. (2011). 'Female Competition and Its Evolutionary Consequences in Mammals'. In: *Biological Reviews*, 86(2): 341–66.
2 Van Schaik, C. & J.B. Silk (2013). 'Contributions of Sarah Blaffer Hrdy'. In: *Evol Anthropol*, 22(5): 200–1.
3 https://www.bbc.co.uk/mediacentre/mediapacks/planet-earth-ii/cities
4 Bethmann, D. et al. (2009). 'Why are More Boys Born During War? Evidence from Germany at Mid Century'. In: Ruhr Economic Papers, 154.
5 Abreu, A.P. & U.B. Kaiser (2016). 'Pubertal development and regulation'. In: *Lancet Diabetes Endocrinol*, Mar; 4(3): 254–64.
6 Carson, R. (1962). *Silent Spring*. Boston: Houghton Mifflin.
7 Kasteren, J. van (1996). 'De kwaliteit van het mannelijk zaad'. https://www.emokennislink.nl
8 Carlsen, E. & N.E. Skakkebaek. (1992). 'Evidence for decreasing quality of semen during past 50 years'. In: *BMJ*, Sept 12; 305(6854): 609–13.
9 Tiegs, A.W. et al. (2019). 'Total Motile Sperm Count Trend Over Time: Evaluation of Semen Analyses from 119,972 Men from Subfertile Couples'. In: *Urology*, Oct; 132: 109–116.
10 Mammi, C. et al. (2012). 'Androgens and adipose tissue in males: a complex and reciprocal interplay'. In: *Int J Endocrinol*: 789653.
11 Levine H. et al. (2017). 'Temporal trends in sperm count: a systematic review and meta-regression analysis'. In: *Hum Reprod Update*, Nov 1; 23(6): 646–59.
12 Zerjal, T. et al. (2003). 'Genetic Legacy of The Mongols'. In: *Am J Hum Genet*, Mar; 72(3): 717–21.
13 Barker, D.J.P., Lampl, M., Roseboom, T. & N. Winder (2012). 'Resource Allocation in Utero and Health in Later Life'. In: *Placenta*, Nov; 33 Suppl 2: e30–4.
14 Lumey, L.H. & A.D. Stein (1997). 'Offspring Birth Weights after Maternal Intrauterine Undernutrition: a Comparison within Sibships'. In: *Am J Epidemiol*, 146(10): 810–9.
15 Ward, Z.J. et al. (2019). 'Projected U.S. State-Level Prevalence of Adult Obesity and Severe Obesity'. In: *N Engl J Med*, Dec 19; 381(25): 2440–50.
16 Han, J. et al. (2005). 'Long-Term Effect of Maternal Obesity on Pancreatic Beta Cells of Offspring: Reduced Beta Cell Adaptation to High Glucose and High-Fat Diet Challenges in Adult Female Mouse Offspring'. In: *Diabetologia*, 48: 1810–18.
17 Gaspar, R.S. et al. (2021). 'Maternal and offspring high-fat diet leads to platelet hyperactivation in male mice offspring'. In: *Scientific Reports*, 11(1473).

18  Rodríguez-González, G.L. et al. (2015). 'Maternal Obesity and
    Overnutrition Increase Oxidative Stress in Male Rat Offspring
    Reproductive System and Decrease Fertility'. In: *International
    Journal of Obesity*; 39: 549–56.
19  Beemsterboer, S.N. (2006). 'The Paradox of Declining Fertility
    but Increasing Twinning Rates with Advance Maternal Age'. In:
    *Human Reproduction*, 21(6): 1531–2.
20  Azziz, R., Dumesic, D.A. & M.O. Goodarzi (2011). 'Polycystic
    ovary syndrome: an ancient disorder?'. In: *Fertil Steril*, 95(5).
21  Kumar, P. et al. (2011). 'Ovarian Hyperstimulation Syndrome'. In:
    *J Hum Reprod Sci*, May–Aug; 4(2): 70–75.
22  Taguchi, O. et al. (1984). 'Timing and Irreversibility of Müllerian
    Duct Inhibition in the Embryonic Reproductive Tract of the
    Human Male'. In: *Developmental Biology*, 106 (2): 394–8.
23  Mauro, S. et al. (2021). 'New Insights into Anti-Müllerian
    Hormone Role in the Hypothalamic-Pituitary-Gonadal Axis and
    Neuroendocrine Development'. In: *Cellular and Molecular Life
    Sciences*, 78: 1–16.
24  Wiweko, B. et al. (2014). 'Anti-Müllerian Hormone as a Diagnostic
    and Prognostic Tool for PCOS Patients'. In: *J Assist Reprod Genet*,
    Oct; 31(10): 1311–16.
25  Oncul, M. (2014). 'May AMH levels distinguish LOCAH from
    PCOS among hirsute women?' In: *Eur Journal of Obstetric Gynecol
    Reprod Biol*, July; 178: 183–7.
26  Pardoe, R. (1988). *The Female Pope; the Mystery of Pope Joan:
    the First Complete Documentation of the Facts Behind the Legend*.
    Wellingborough: Crucible.
27  New, M.I., Kitzinger, E.S. (1993). 'Pope Joan: a recognizable
    syndrome'. In: *J Clin Endocrinol Metab*, Jan; 76(1): 3–13.
28  Speiser, P.W. (1985). 'High frequency of nonclassical steroid 21-
    hydroxylase deficiency'. In: *Am J Hum Genet*, July; 37(4): 650–67.
29  Yaron, Y. et al. (2002). 'Maternal Serum HCG is Higher in the
    Presence of a Female Fetus as Early as Week 3 Post-Fertilization'.
    In: *Human Reprod*, Feb; 17(2): 485–9.
30  Lee, N. et al. (2011). 'Nausea and Vomiting of Pregnancy'. In:
    *Gastroenterol Clin North Am*, Jun; 40(2): 309–34, vii.
31  Buckwalter J.G. (1999). 'Pregnancy, the Postpartum, and
    Steroid Hormones: Effects on Cognition and Mood'. In:
    *Psychoneuroendocrinology*, Jan; 24(1): 69–84.
32  https://en.wikipedia.org/wiki/The_Distaff_Gospels
33  McFadzen, M. et al. (2017). 'Maternal Intuition of Fetal Gender'.
    In: *J Patient Cent Res Rev*, Summer; 4(3): 125–130.
34  https://www.sciencedirect.com/topics/veterinary-science-and-
    veterinary-medicine/human-placental-lactogen
35  Abu-Raya, B. et al. (2020). 'Maternal Immunological Adaptation
    During Normal Pregnancy'. In: *Front. Immunol*, 7 Oct: 11:575197.

36 https://www.sciencedirect.com/science/article/abs/pii/ S0301211520304334

37 Keynes, M. (2000). 'The aching head and increasing blindness of Queen Mary I'. In: *Med Biogr*, May; 8(2): 102–9.

38 Deelen, M. (2020). 'Melk van allebei je moeders, dat kan dus ook'. In: *de Volkskrant*, 5 June.

39 Guastellaa, A.J. et al. (2010). 'Intranasal Oxytocin Improves Emotion Recognition for Youth with Autism Spectrum Disorders'. In: *Biological Psychiatry*, 67(7): 692–4.

40 Swaab, D.F., Boer, G.J., Boer, K., Dogterom, J., Van Leeuwen, F.W. & M.Visser (1978). 'Fetal neuroendocrine mechanisms in development and parturition'. In: *Prog Brain Res*, 48: 277–90.

41 Bell, A.F. et al. (2014). 'Beyond Labor: the Role of Natural and Synthetic Oxytocin in the Transition to Motherhood'. In: *J Midwifery Womens Health*, Jan–Feb; 59(1): 35–42.

42 Carvalho, B. et al. (2006). 'Experimental heat pain for detecting pregnancy-induced analgesia in humans'. In: Anesthesia & Analgesia, 103(5): 1283–7.

43 Knechtle, B. et al. (2018). 'Physiology and Pathophysiology in Ultra-Marathon Running'. In: *Front Physiol*, Jun 1; 9: 634.

44 https://en.wikipedia.org/wiki/Ebers_Papyrus

45 https://www.ncbi.nlm.nih.gov/books/NBK53528/

46 Strandwitz, P. (2018). 'Neurotransmitter Modulation by the Gut Microbiota'. In: *Brain Res*, Aug 15; 1693(Pt B): 128–33.

47 Schulte, E.M. et al. (2015). 'Which Foods May Be Addictive? The Roles of Processing, Fat Content, and Glycemic Load'. In: *PLoS One*, Feb 18; 10(2): e0117959.

48 Tasca, C. et al. (2012). 'Women and Hysteria in the History of Mental Health'. In: *Clin Pract Epidemiol Ment Health*, 8: 110–119.

49 Maines, R.P. (1998). *The Technology of Orgasm: 'Hysteria', the Vibrator, and Women's Sexual Satisfaction*. Baltimore: Johns Hopkins University Press.

50 Anders, S.M. van (2009). 'Associations among physiological and subjective sexual response, sexual desire, and salivary steroid hormones in healthy premenopausal women'. In: *J Sex Med*, Mar; 6(3): 739–51.

51 Stevenson, S. & J. Tornton (2007). 'Effect of estrogens on skin aging and the potential role of SERMS'. In: *Clin Interv Aging*, Sept; 2(3): 283–97.

52 Munn, D.H. et al. (1998). 'Prevention of Allogeneic Fetal Rejection by Tryptophan Catabolism'. In: *Science*, Aug 21; 281(5380): 1191–3.

53 Russo, S. et al. (2009). 'Tryptophan as an Evolutionarily Conserved Signal to Brain Serotonin: Molecular Evidence and Psychiatric Implications'. In: *World J Biol Psychiatry*; 10(4): 258–68.

54 Høgh, S., Hegaard, H.K., Renault, K.M. et al. (2021). 'Short-Term

Oestrogen as a Strategy to Prevent Postpartum Depression in
High-Risk Women: Protocol for the Double-Blind, Randomised,
Placebo-Controlled MAMA Clinical Trial'. In: *BMJ Open*, 11:
e052922.

55  Edelstein, R.S. et al. (2015). 'Prenatal hormones in first-time
expectant parents: Longitudinal changes and within-couple
correlations'. In: *Am J Hum Biol*, May–Jun; 27(3): 317–25.

56  Li, T. et al. (2017). 'Intranasal oxytocin, but not vasopressin,
augments neural responses to toddlers in human fathers'. In:
*Horm Behav*, July; 93: 193–202.

57  Mascaro, J.S., Hackett, P.D. & J.K. Rilling (2014). 'Differential
neural responses to child and sexual stimuli in human
fathers and non-fathers and their hormonal correlates'. In:
*Psychoneuroendocrinology*, Aug; 46: 153–63.

58  Gettler, L.T. et al. (2011). 'Longitudinal evidence that fatherhood
decreases testosterone in human males'. In: *PNAS*, 108 (39):
16194–9.

59  Fleming, A.S. et al. (2002). 'Testosterone and prolactin are
associated with emotional responses to infant cries in new
fathers'. In: *Hormones and Behavior*, 42(4): 399–413. See also:
https://pubmed.ncbi.nlm.nih.gov/25504668/

60  Masoni, S. et al. (1994). 'The couvade syndrome'. In: *Psychosom
Obstet Gynaecol*, Sept; 15(3): 125–31.

61  Miller, S.L. & J.K. Maner (2010). 'Scent of a woman: men's
testosterone responses to olfactory ovulation cues'. In: *Psychol Sci*,
21(2): 276–83.

62  http://en.antiquitatem.com/couvade-matriarchy-gynecocracy-
apolloniu, and https://en.wikipedia.org/wiki/Couvade

63  Cohn, B.A. (1994). 'In search of human skin pheromones'. In:
*Arch Dermatol*, 130 (8): 1048–51.

64  Trotier, D. (2011). 'Vomeronasal organ and human pheromones'.
In: *Eur Ann Otorhinolaryngol Head Neck Dis*, Sept; 128(4): 184–90.

65  Keverne, E.B. (1999). 'The vomeronasal organ'. In: *Science*, Oct 22;
286(5440): 716–20.

66  Stoyanov, G., Moneva, K., Sapundzhiev, N. & A.B. Tonchev
(2016). 'The vomeronasal organ – incidence in a Bulgarian
population'. In: *Journal of Laryngology and Otology*, 130 (4): 344–7.

67  Verhaeghe, J. et al. (2013). 'Pheromones and their effect on
women's mood and sexuality'. In: *Facts Views. Vis Obgyn*, 5(3):
189–95.

68  Miller, G. (2007). 'Ovulatory cycle effects on tip earnings by lap
dancers: Economic evidence for human estrus?'. In: *Evolution and
Human Behavior*, 28: 375–81.

69  https://healthland.time.com/2011/09/13/
why-do-dads-have-lower-levels-of-testosterone/

70  https://en.wikipedia.org/wiki/Coolidge_effect

71 Pizzari, T. et al. (2003). 'Sophisticated Sperm Allocation in Male Fowl'. In: *Nature*, 426: 70–74.
72 Fiorino, D.F., Coury, A. & A. G. Phillips (1997). 'Dynamic Changes in Nucleus Accumbens Dopamine Efflux During the Coolidge Effect in Male Rats'. In: *Journal of Neuroscience*, 17(12): 4849–55.

## Chapter 2 – The Big Run-up

1 Hompes, T. et al. (2013). 'Investigating the influence of maternal cortisol and emotional state during pregnancy on the DNA methylation status of the glucocorticoid receptor gene (NR3C1) promoter region in cord blood'. In: *Journal of Psychiatric Research*, July; 47(7): 880–91.
2 Radtke, K.M. et al. (2015). 'Epigenetic Modifications of the Glucocorticoid Receptor Gene Are Associated with the Vulnerability to Psychopathology in Childhood Maltreatment'. In: *Translational Psychiatry*, 5: e571.
3 Hansen, D. et al. (2000). 'Serious Life Events and Congenital Malformations: a National Study with Complete Follow-Up'. In: *Lancet*, Sept 9; 356(9233): 875–80. doi: 10.1016/S0140–6736(00)02676–3.
4 Laplante, D.P. et al. (2004). 'Stress During Pregnancy Affects General Intellectual and Language Functioning in Human Toddlers'. In: *Pediatric Research*, 56: 400–410.
5 https://www.nobelprize.org/prizes/medicine/1977/summary/
6 Forest, M.G. et al. (1973). 'Total and Unbound Testosterone Levels in the Newborn and in Normal and Hypogonadal Children: Use of a Sensitive Radioimmunoassay for Testosterone'. In: *J Clin Endocrinol Metab*, Jun; 36(6): 1132–42.
7 Forest, M.G., Sizonenko, P.C., Cathiard, A.M. & J. Bertrand (1974). 'Hypophyso-Gonadal Function in Humans During the First Year of Life. 1 Evidence for Testicular Activity in Early Infancy'. In: *J Clin Invest*, Mar; 53(3): 819–28.
8 Andersson, A.M. et al. (1998). 'Longitudinal Reproductive Hormone Profiles in Infants: Peak of Inhibin B Levels in Infant Boys Exceeds Levels in Adult Men'. In: *J Clin Endocrinol Metab*, Feb; 83(2): 675–81.
9 François, C.M. et al. (2017). 'A Novel Action of Follicle-Stimulating Hormone in the Ovary Promotes Estradiol Production Without Inducing Excessive Follicular Growth Before Puberty'. In: *Sci Rep*, Apr 11; 7: 46222.
10 https://www.ncj.nl/richtlijnen/alle-richtlijnen/richtlijn/?richtlijn=2&rlpag=378
11 Sømod, M.E. et al. (2016). 'Increasing incidence of premature

thelarche in the Central Region of Denmark – Challenges in differentiating girls less than 7 years of age with premature thelarche from girls with precocious puberty in real-life practice'. In: *Pediatric Endocrinology*, 2016(4).

12  Kinson, G.A. (1976). 'Pineal factors in the control of testicular function'. In: *Adv Sex Horm Res*, 2: 87–139.

13  Descartes, R. (1664). *Traité de l'homme*. Paris: Charles Angot.

14  Partsch, C.J. & W.G. Sippell (2001). 'Pathogenesis and epidemiology of precocious puberty. Effects of exogenous oestrogens'. In: *Hum Reprod Update*, May–Jun; 7(3): 292–302.

15  https://www.dailymail.co.uk/femail/article-508020/The-girls-started-going-puberty-three.html

16  Okdemir, D. et al. (2014). 'Premature thelarche related to fennel tea consumption?'. In: *J Pediatr Endocr Met*, 27(1–2): 1759.

17  https://onlinelibrary.wiley.com/doi/full/10.1111/jpc.12837

18  Zung, A. (2008). 'Breast Development in the First 2 Years of Life: an Association with Soy-Based Infant Formulas'. In: *Pediatr Gastroenterol Nutr*, Feb; 46(2): 191–5.

19  Andersson, A.M. & N.E. Skakkebaek. (1999). 'Exposure to exogenous estrogens in food: possible impact on human development and health'. In: *Eur J Endocrinol*, Jun; 140(6): 477–85.

20  Sáenz De Rodríguez, C. & M. Toro-Solá (1982). 'Anabolic Steroids in Meat and Premature Thelarche'. In: *Lancet*, 319(8284): 1300.

21  Pérez Comas, A. (1982). 'Precocious Sexual Development in Puerto Rico'. In: *Lancet*, 319(8284): 1299–1300; Loizzo, A. et al. (1984). 'The Case of Diethylstilbestrol Treated Veal Contained in Homogenized Baby-Foods in Italy. Methodological and Toxicological Aspects'. In: *Ann Ist Super Sanita*, Vol. 20, N. 2–3, 215–20.

22  Gaspari, L., Morcrette, E., Jeandel, C., Valé, F.D, Paris, F. & C. Sultan (2014). 'Dramatic Rise in the Prevalence of Precocious Puberty in Girls over the Past 20 Years in the South of France'. In: *Horm Res Ped*; 82 suppl. 1: 291–2.

23  https://www.rivm.nl/en/news/dutch-people-eat-more-healthy-foods-more-plant-products-less-red-and-processed-meat-0

24  Hoffman, J.R. & M.J. Falvo (2004). 'Protein – Which is Best?'. In: *J Sports Sci Med*, 3, 118–30.

25  Barrett, J.R. (2002). 'Soy and children's health: a formula for trouble'. In: *Environ Health Perspect*, Jun; 110(6): A294–6.

26  Strom, B.L. et al. (2001). 'Exposure to soy-based formula in infancy and endocrinological and reproductive outcomes in young adulthood'. In: *JAMA*, Aug 15; 286(7): 807–14.

27  Colborn, T. (1990). *Great Lakes, Great Legacy?* Institute for Research and Public Policy.

28  Gaspari, L. (2012). 'High Prevalence of Micropenis in 2710 Male Newborns from an Intensive-Use Pesticide Area of Northeastern Brazil'. In: *Int J Androl*, Jun; 35(3): 253–64.

29  https://en.wikipedia.org/wiki/Scoubidou
30  Paris, F. et al. (2013). 'Increased serum estrogenic bioactivity in girls with premature thelarche: a marker of environmental pollutant exposure?'. In: *Gynecol Endocrinol*, Aug; 29(8): 788–92.
31  Gaspari, L. (2011). 'Peripheral precocious puberty in a 4-month-old girl: role of pesticides?'. In: *Gynecol Endocrinol*, Sept; 27(9): 721–4.
32  Vogiatzi, M.G. et al. (2016). 'Menstrual Bleeding as a Manifestation of Mini-Puberty of Infancy in Severe Prematurity'. In: *J Pediatr*, Nov; 178: 292–5.
33  Mendez, M.A. et al. (2002). 'Soy-based formulae and infant growth and development: a review'. In: *J Nutr*, Aug; 132(8): 2127–30.
34  Thorup, J. et al. (2010). 'What is new in cryptorchidism and hypospadias – a critical review on the testicular dysgenesis hypothesis'. In: *J Pediatr Surg*, Oct; 45(10): 2074–86.
35  https://allthatsinteresting.com/annie-jones-bearded-lady
36  https://isgeschiedenis.nl/nieuws/julia-pastrana-de-mexicaanse-aapvrouw
37  https://en.wikipedia.org/wiki/Krao_Farini
38  The L.A. Circus Congress of Freaks and Exotics.
39  See Instagram: Rose Geil, Harnaam Kaur.
40  Fawzy, F. et al. (2015). 'Cryptorchidism and Fertility'. In: *Clin Med Insights Reprod Health*, Dec; 9: 39–43.
41  Gill, W.B. (1988). 'Effects on Human Males of in Utero Exposure to Exogenous Sex Hormones'. In: Mori, T. & H. Nagasawa (Eds.), *Toxicity of Hormones in Perinatal Life*. Boca Raton: CRC Press Inc., 161–77.
42  https://historiek.net/testikel/64849/
43  Ford, B. (2011). *Secret Weapons: Technology, Science and the Race to Win World War II*. Bloomsbury Publishing Plc.
44  Brucker-Davis, F. et al. (2003). 'Update on cryptorchidism: endocrine, environmental and therapeutic aspects'. In: *J Endocrinol Invest*, Jun; 26(6): 575–87.
45  García-Rodríguez, F. et al. (1996). 'Exposure to pesticides and cryptorchidism: geographical evidence of a possible association'. In: *Environ Health Perspect*, Oct; 104(10): 1090–5.
46  Imajima, T. et al. (1997). 'Prenatal phthalate causes cryptorchidism postnatally by inducing transabdominal ascent of the testis in fetal rats'. In: *J Pediatr Surg*, Jan; 32(1): 18–21.
47  Hadziselimovic, F. et al. (2005). 'The importance of mini-puberty for fertility in cryptorchidism'. In: *Journal of Urology*, 174: 1536–9.
48  Zhang, R., et al. (2002). 'A quantitative (stereological) study of the effects of experimental unilateral cryptorchidism and subsequent orchiopexy on spermatogenesis in adult rabbit testis'. In: *Reproduction*, 124(1): 95–105.

49 Moon, J. et al. (2014). 'Unilateral cryptorchidism induces morphological changes of testes and hyperplasia of Sertoli cells in a dog'. In: *Lab Anim Res*, Dec; 30(4): 185–9.

50 Verkauskas, G. et al. (2016). 'Prospective study of histological and endocrine parameters of gonadal function in boys with cryptorchidism'. In: *J Pediatr Urol*, Aug; 12(4): 238.e1–6.

51 Boas, M. et al. (2006). 'Postnatal penile length and growth rate correlate to serum testosterone levels: a longitudinal study of 1962 normal boys'. In: *Eur J Endocrinol*, Jan; 154(1): 125–9.

52 Koskenniemi, J. et al. (2018). 'Postnatal Changes in Testicular Position Are Associated With IGF-I and Function of Sertoli and Leydig Cells'. In: *J Clin Endocrinol Metab*, Apr 1; 103(4): 1429–37.

53 Bin-Abbas, B. et al. (1999). 'Congenital hypogonadotropic hypogonadism and micropenis: effect of testosterone treatment on adult penile size – Why sex reversal is not indicated'. In: *J Pediatr*, May; 134(5): 579–83.

54 Reiner, W.G. et al. (2004). 'Discordant sexual identity in some genetic males with cloacal exstrophy assigned to female sex at birth'. In: *N Engl J Med*, Jan 22; 350(4): 333–41.

55 Reiner, W.G. (2005). 'Gender identity and sex-of-rearing in children with disorders of sexual differentiation'. In: *J Pediatr Endocrinol Metab*, Jun; 18(6): 549–53.

56 Hines, M. et al. (2015). 'Early androgen exposure and human gender development'. In: Biol Sex Differ, Feb 26; 6(3).

57 https://en.wikipedia.org/wiki/Foekje_Dillema

58 Dohle, M.J.M. (2008). *Het verwoeste leven van Foekje Dillema*. Amsterdam: De Arbeiderspers.

59 https://www.npostart.nl/andere-tijden-sport/29-07-2018/vpwon_1293632

60 See note 57.

61 Stiles, J. et al. (2010). 'The basics of brain development'. In: *Neuropsychol Rev*, Dec; 20(4): 327–48.

62 Hines, M. et al. (2016). 'The early postnatal period, mini-puberty, provides a window on the role of testosterone in human neurobehavioural development'. In: *Current Opinion in Neurobiology*, 38: 69–73.

63 Swaab, D. (2010). *Wij zijn ons brein. Van baarmoeder tot alzheimer*. Amsterdam: Contact.

64 Pasterski, V.L. et al. (2005). 'Prenatal hormones and postnatal socialization by parents as determinants of male-typical toy play in girls with congenital adrenal hyperplasia'. In: *Child Dev*, Jan–Feb; 76(1): 264–78.

65 Lamminmaki, A. et al. (2012). 'Testosterone measured in infancy predicts subsequent sex-typed behavior in boys and in girls'. In: *Hormones and Behavior*, 61: 611–16.

66 Pasterski, V.L. et al. (2015). 'Postnatal penile growth concurrent

with mini-puberty predicts later sex-typed play behavior: Evidence for neurobehavioral effects of the postnatal androgen surge in typically developing boys'. In: *Hormones and Behavior*, 69: 98–105.

67   Wallen, K. (1996). 'Nature needs nurture: the interaction of hormonal and social influences on the development of behavioral sex differences in rhesus monkeys'. In: *Hormones and Behavior*, 30(4): 364–78.

68   Morgan, K. et al. (2011). 'The sex bias in novelty preference of preadolescent mouse pups may require testicular Müllerian inhibiting substance'. In: *Behav Brain Res*, Aug 1; 221(1): 304–6.

69   Golombok, S. & J. Rust (1993). 'The Measurement of Gender Role Behaviour in Pre-School Children: a Research Note'. In: *Journal of Child Psychology and Psychiatry*, 34(5): 805–11.

70   Alexander, G. (2014). 'Postnatal testosterone concentrations and male social development'. In: *Front Endocrinol (Lausanne)*, Feb 21; 5: 15.

71   Pankhurst, M.W. et al. (2012). 'Inhibin B and anti-Müllerian hormone/Müllerian-inhibiting substance may contribute to the male bias in autism'. In: *Transl Psychiatry*, Aug 14; 2(8): e148.

72   Hadziselimovic, F. et al. (2014). 'Decreased expression of genes associated with memory and x-linked mental retardation in boys with non-syndromic cryptorchidism and high infertility risk'. In: *Mol Syndromol*, Feb; 5(2): 76–80.

73   Hadziselimovic, F. et al. (2017). 'Genes Involved in Long-Term Memory Are Expressed in Testis of Cryptorchid Boys and Respond to GnRHA Treatment'. In: *Cytogenet Genome Res*, 152(1): 9–15.

74   Schaadt, G. et al. (2015). 'Sex hormones in early infancy seem to predict aspects of later language development'. In: *Brain Language*, 141: 70–76.

75   Hier D.B. & W.F. Crowley (1982). 'Spatial ability in androgen-deficient men'. In: *N Engl J Med*, 306: 1202–5

## Chapter 3 – Growing Pains and Butterflies

1   Hall, G.S. (1904). *Adolescence: Its Psychology and Its Relations to Physiology, Anthropology, Sociology, Sex, Crime, Religion and Education*. New York: D. Appleton & Company.

2   https://www.theguardian.com/society/2012/oct/21/puberty-adolescence-childhood-onset

3   Euling, S.Y. et al. (2008). 'Examination of US puberty-timing data from 1940 to 1994 for secular trends: panel fndings'. In: *Pediatrics*, Feb; 121 Suppl 3: S172–91.

4   Lee, J.M. et al. (2016). 'Timing of Puberty in Overweight Versus Obese Boys'. In: *Pediatrics*, Feb; 137(2): e20150164.

# Notes

5   Tanner, J.M. (2010). *A History of the Study of Human Growth*.
    Cambridge University Press.
6   https://en.wikipedia.org/wiki/Parts_of_Animals
7   Rall, G.F. (1669). *De generatione animalium disquisitio medico-
    physica in qua celeberrimorum virorum*. Frankfurt: Melchior
    Klosemann: 164–5.
8   Protsiv, M. et al, (2020). 'Decreasing human body temperature in
    the United States since the industrial revolution'. In: *eLife*, Jan 7;
    9:e 49555.
9   Janssen, D.F. (2021). 'Puer Barbatus: Precocious Puberty in Early
    Modern Medicine'. In: *Journal of the History of Medicine and Allied
    Sciences*, Jan; 76(1): 20–52.
10  https://www.nrc.nl/nieuws/2008/03/22/
    ik-ruik-seks-11508699-a160883
11  McClintock, M.K. (1971). 'Menstrual Synchrony and Suppression'.
    In: *Nature*, 229(5282): 244–5.
12  Stern, K. & M.K. McClintock (1998). 'Regulation of Ovulation by
    Human Pheromones'. In: *Nature*, 392(6672): 177–9.
13  Shinohara, K. et al. (2001). 'Axillary Pheromones Modulate
    Pulsatile LH Secretion in Humans'. In: *Neuroreport*, 12(5): 893–5.
14  Daw, S.F. (1970). 'Age of Boys' Puberty in Leipzig, 1727–49, as
    Indicated by Voice Breaking in J. S. Bach's Choir Members'.
    *Human Biology*, 42(1): 87–9.
15  https://www.jellejolles.nl/kennisarchief/boeken/tienerbrein/
16  Crone, E. et al. (2018). 'Media use and brain development during
    adolescence'. In: *Nat Commun*, 9: 588.
17  Spielberg, J.M. et al. (2015). 'Pubertal testosterone influences
    threat-related amygdala-orbitofrontal cortex coupling'. In: *Soc
    Cogn Affect Neurosci*, Mar; 10(3): 408–15.
18  Cardoos, S.L. et al. (2017). 'Social status strategy in early
    adolescent girls: Testosterone and value-based decision making'.
    In: *Psychoneuroendocrinology*, 81: 14–21.
19  Nave, G. et al. (2017). 'Single-Dose Testosterone Administration
    Impairs Cognitive Reflection in Men'. In: *Psychol Sci*, 28(10):
    1398–1407.
20  Chicaiza-Becerra, L., Garcia-Molina, M. et al. (2017). 'Prenatal
    testosterone predicts financial risk taking: Evidence from Latin
    America'. In: *Personality and Individual Differences*, 116: 32–7.
21  https://en.wikipedia.org/wiki/Coming_of_Age_in_Samoa
22  Bourbon, N. (Cratander 1533). *Nugae (Bagatelles)*. Reprint Librarie
    Droz; Bilingual edition (31 Dec. 2008).
23  Goleman, D. (1996). *Emotionele intelligentie*. Amsterdam: Contact.
24  Shoda, Y. & W.D. Mischel (1990). 'Predicting Adolescent
    Cognitive and Self-Regulatory Competencies From Preschool
    Delay of Gratification: Identifying Diagnostic Conditions'. In:
    *Developmental Psychology*, 26(6): 978–86.

25 Watts, T.W. et al. (2018). 'Revisiting the Marshmallow Test: A Conceptual Replication Investigating Links Between Early Delay of Gratification and Later Outcomes'. In: *Psychol Sci*, July; 29(7): 1159–77.

26 Harris, C. et al. (2015). 'Changes in dietary intake during puberty and their determinants: results from the GINIplus birth cohort study'. In: *BMC Public Health*, Sept 2; 15: 841.

27 Terry, N. and K.G. Margolis (2017). 'Serotonergic Mechanisms Regulating the GI Tract: Experimental Evidence and Therapeutic Relevance'. In: *Handb Exp Pharmacol*, 239: 319–342.

28 Pease, A. (1999). *Waarom mannen niet luisteren en vrouwen niet kunnen kaartlezen*. Utrecht: Het Spectrum.

29 Graf, H. et al. (2019). 'Serotonergic, Dopaminergic, and Noradrenergic Modulation of Erotic Stimulus Processing in the Male Human Brain'. In: *J Clin Med*, Mar; 8(3): 363.

30 Hughes, S.M. et al. (2007). 'Sex differences in romantic kissing among college students: An evolutionary perspective'. In: *Evolutionary Psychology*, 5(3): 612–31.

31 Wlodarski, R. et al. (2014). 'What's in a Kiss? The Effect of Romantic Kissing on Mate Desirability'. In: *Evolutionary Psychology*, 12(1): 178–99.

32 Prosser, C.G. et al. (1983). 'Saliva and breast milk composition during the menstrual cycle of women'. In: *Aust J Exp Biol Med Sci*, Jun; 61 (Pt 3): 265–75.

33 Cerda-Molina, A.L. et al. (2013). 'Changes in Men's Salivary Testosterone and Cortisol Levels, and in Sexual Desire after Smelling Female Axillary and Vulvar Scents'. In: *Front Endocrinol (Lausanne)*, Oct 28; 4: 159.

34 Kromer, J. et al. (2016). 'Influence of HLA on human partnership and sexual satisfaction'. In: *Sci Rep*, 6: 32550.

35 Roberts, S.C. et al. (2008). 'MHC-correlated odour preferences in humans and the use of oral contraceptives'. In: *Proc Biol Sci*, Dec 7; 275(1652): 2715–22.

36 https://www.theguardian.com/lifeandstyle/2013/sep/08/can-you-smell-perfect-partner

37 https://www.latimes.com/archives/la-xpm-1987-12-02-mn-17142-story.html

38 Ranke, M.B. et al. (2018). 'Growth hormone – past, present and future'. In: *Nat Rev Endocrinol*, May; 14(5): 285–300.

39 https://www.nemokennislink.nl/publicaties/waarom-nederlanders-zolang-zijn/

40 Rich-Edwards, J.W. (2007). 'Milk consumption and the prepubertal somatotropic axis'. In: *Nutr J*, Sept 27; 6: 28.

41 https://rarediseases.org/rare-diseases/acromegaly/

42 https://en.wikipedia.org/wiki/Periplus

43 Armocida, E. et al. (2020). 'Hereditary acromegalic gigantism

in the family of Roman Emperor Maximinus Trax'. In: *Med Hypotheses*, Mar; 136: 109525.

44 Minozzi, S. et al. (2012). 'Pituitary disease from the past: a rare case of gigantism in skeletal remains from the Roman Imperial Age'. In: *J Clin Endocrinol Metab*, Dec; 97(12): 4302–3.

45 Chahal, H.S. et al. (2011). 'AIP mutation in pituitary adenomas in the 18th century and today'. In: *N Engl J Med*, Jan 6; 364(1): 43–50.

46 https://en.wikipedia.org/wiki/Trijntje_Keever

47 Herder, W.W. de, (2004). 'Giantism. A historical and medical view'. In: *Ned Tijdschr Geneeskd*, Dec 25; 148(52): 2585–90.

48 https://en.wikipedia.org/wiki/Potsdam_Giants

49 LeBourgeois, M.K. et al. (2017). 'Digital Media and Sleep in Childhood and Adolescence'. In: *Pediatrics*, Nov; 140 (Suppl 2): S92–6.

50 Valcavi, R. et al. (1993). 'Melatonin stimulates growth hormone secretion through pathways other than the growth hormone-releasing hormone'. In: *Clin Endocrinol (Oxf)*, Aug; 39(2): 193–9.

51 https://www.cbs.nl/nl-nl/nieuws/2021/37/nederlanders-korter-maar-nogsteeds-lang

52 Wideman, L. et al. (2002). 'Growth hormone release during acute and chronic aerobic and resistance exercise: recent findings'. In: *Sports Med*, 32(15): 987–1004.

53 https://www.medicosport.eu/nl/doping/doping1996-os.html

54 Ho, K.Y. et al. (1988). 'Fasting enhances growth hormone secretion and amplifies the complex rhythms of growth hormone secretion in man'. In: *J Clin Invest*, Apr; 81(4): 968–75.

55 Boudesteyn, K. et al. (2002). 'Ghrelin, an important hormone produced by the stomach'. In: *Ned Tijdschr Geneeskd*, Oct 12; 146(41): 1929–33.

56 Levy, E. et al. (2019). 'Intermittent Fasting and Its Effects on Athletic Performance: A Review'. In: *Curr Sports Med Rep*, July; 18(7): 266–9.

57 Schorr, M. et al. (2017). 'The endocrine manifestations of anorexia nervosa: mechanisms and management'. In: *Nat Rev Endocrinol*, Mar; 13(3): 174–86.

58 Muñoz-Hoyos, A. et al. (2011). 'Psychosocial dwarfism: psychopathological aspects and putative neuroendocrine markers'. In: *Psychiatry Res*, Jun 30; 188(1): 96–101.

59 Gohlke, B.C., Frazer, F.L. & R. Stanhope (2004). 'Growth hormone secretion and long-term growth data in children with psychosocial short stature treated by different changes in environment'. In: *J Pediatr Endocrinol Metab*, 17(4): 637–43.

60 Powell-Jackson, J. et al. (1985). 'Creutzfeldt-Jakob disease after administration of human growth hormone'. In: *Lancet*, Aug 3; 2(8449): 244–6.

## Chapter 4 – Homosexuality and Transgender People

1  https://www.boomgeschiedenis.nl/
   product/100-3527_Transgender-in-Nederland
2  Money, J. et al. (1955). 'An examination of some basic sexual
   concepts: the evidence of human hermaphroditism'. In: *Bulletin
   of the Johns Hopkins Hospital*, 97(4): 301–19.
3  Dohle, M.J.M. (2008). *Het verwoeste leven van Foekje Dillema*.
   Amsterdam: De Arbeiderspers.
4  https://www.cbc.ca/news/world/gay-penguin-couple-adopts-
   abandoned-egg-in-german-zoo-1.794702
5  http://www.bbc.com/earth/
   story/20150206-are-there-any-homosexual-animals
6  https://en.wikipedia.org/wiki/Hermaphrodite
7  https://natuurwijzer.naturalis.nl/leerobjecten/
   soms-een-man-soms-een-vrouw
8  Spencer-Hall, A. and B. Gutt. (2021). *Trans and Genderqueer
   Subjects in Medieval Hagiography*. Amsterdam: Amsterdam
   University Press.
9  Herman, J.L. et al. (2017). 'Demographic and Health
   Characteristics of Transgender Adults in California: Findings
   from the 2015–2016 California Health Interview Survey'. In:
   *Policy Brief (UCLA Center for Health Policy Research)*, Oct 1; 1: 1–10.
10  https://williamsinstitute.law.ucla.edu/publications/
    global-acceptance-index-lgbt/
11  https://www.ad.nl/show/nikkie-de-jager-dacht-na-coming-out-
    dat-alles-voorbij-was~abd09f3e/?referrer=https%3A%2F%2Fwww.
    google.nl%2F
12  https://www.scp.nl/publicaties/monitors/2018/11/21/
    lhbt-monitor-2018
13  https://www.smithsonianmag.com/arts-culture/
    when-did-girls-start-wearing-pink-1370097/
14  https://en.wikipedia.org/wiki/Mamie_Eisenhower
15  Jonauskaite, D. et al. (2019). 'Pink for girls, red for boys, and blue
    for both genders: Colour preferences in children and adults'. In:
    *Sex Roles*, 80: 630–642.
16  https://de.wikipedia.org/wiki/Das_lila_Lied
17  https://nos.nl/artikel/2193985-best-wel-stoer-meisje-blij-met-
    gendervrije-kleren-bij-hema
18  Vries, A.L.C. de et al (2014). 'Young adult psychological outcome
    after puberty suppression and gender reassignment'. In:
    *Pediatrics*, Oct; 134(4): 696–704.
19  Seibel, B.L. et al. (2018). 'The Impact of the Parental Support on
    Risk Factors in the Process of Gender Affirmation of Transgender
    and Gender Diverse People'. In: *Front Psychol*, Mar 27; 9: 399.
20  Beusekom G. van et al. (2015). 'Same-sex attraction, gender

# Notes

nonconformity, and mental health: The protective role of parental acceptance'. In: *Psychology of Sexual Orientation and Gender Diversity*, 2(3): 307–12.

21  https://en.wikipedia.org/wiki/Elagabalus

22  https://www.ranker.com/list/transgender-people-in-history/devon-ashby

23  The story is told in the film *The Danish Girl* (2016), directed by Tom Hooper, based on the novel of the same name by David Ebershoff, and is sometimes far-fetched.

24  https://en.wikipedia.org/wiki/Christine_Jorgensen

25  Hamburger, C. (1953). 'The desire for change of sex as shown by personal letters from 465 men and women'. In: *Acta Endocrinol (Copenh)*, Dec; 14(4): 361–75.

26  Zhou, J.N. et al. (1995). 'A sex difference in the human brain and its relation to transsexuality'. In: *Nature*, Nov 2; 378(6552): 68–70.

27  https://www.volkskrant.nl/nieuws-achtergrond/het-grootste-compliment-is-ik-heb-een-gewoon-leven-nu~b319de37/

28  https://nos.nl/artikel/2172194-steeds-meer-mensen-wijzigen-hun-geslacht-na-transgenderwet.html

29  https://www.scp.nl/publicaties/publicaties/2017/05/09/transgender-personen-in-nederland

30  Heijer, M. den, et al. (2017). 'Long term hormonal treatment for transgender people'. In: *BMJ*, 359: j5027.

31  https://www.zilverencamera.nl/jaargang/zc-2018/documentair-nationaal-serie/inner-journey-into-manhood/

32  Lo Galbo, C. (2015). 'Ik ben geen George Clooney, maar ik kan ermee door.' Interview with Maxim Februari in *Vrij Nederland*; Februari, M. (2015). *The Making of a Man: Notes on Transsexuality*. Amsterdam: Reaktion.

33  Waanders. L. (2014). Recensie: *De maakbare man: notities over transseksualiteit – Maxim Februari*. Hanta.nl

34  Ongenae, C. (2015). 'Na de geslachtsverandering: Maxim Februari vertelt wat je wel en niet moet weten over transgenders'. Interview at www.catherineongenae.com.

35  Februari, M. (1989). *De zonen van het uitzicht*. Amsterdam: Querido.

36  Swaab, D. & E. Fliers (1985). 'A sexually dimorphic nucleus in the human brain'. In: *Science*, May 31; 228(4703): 1112–5.

37  Swaab, D.F. & M.A. Hofman (1990). 'An enlarged suprachiasmatic nucleus in homosexual men'. In: *Brain Res*, 537(1–2): 141–8.

38  Savic, I., Berglund, H. & P. Lindstrom (2005). 'Brain response to putative pheromones in homosexual men'. In: *Proc Natl Acad Sci USA*, 102: 7356–6.

39  Berglund, H., Lindström, P. & I. Savic (2006). 'Brain response to putative pheromones in lesbian women'. In: *Proc Natl Acad Sci USA*, 103(21): 8269–74.

40 Zhou W, et al. (2014). 'Chemosensory communication of gender through two human steroids in a sexually dimorphic manner'. In: *Curr Biol*, 24(10): 1091–5.

41 Jordan-Young, R. (2011). *Brain Storm: The Flaws in the Science of Sex Differences*. Cambridge: Harvard University Press.

42 Ward, I.L. (1972). 'Prenatal stress feminizes and demasculinizes the behavior of males'. In: *Science*, Jan 7; 175(4017): 82–4.

43 Radtke, K.M. et al. (2015). 'Epigenetic modifications of the glucocorticoid receptor gene are associated with the vulnerability to psychopathology in childhood maltreatment'. In: *Transl Psychiatry*, 5: e571.

44 Waal F., de (2022). *Anders: Gender door de ogen van een primatoloog*. Amsterdam: Pluim.

45 Balthazart, J. (2012). *The Biology of Homosexuality*. Oxford University Press.

46 Terman, L.M. & C.C. Miles (1936). *Sex and Personality: Studies in Masculinity and Femininity*. New York: McGraw-Hill.

47 Blanchard, R.J. (2004). 'Quantitative and theoretical analyses of the relation between older brothers and homosexuality in men'. In: *Theor Biol*, 230(2): 173–187.

48 Blanchard, R. (2008). 'Review and Theory of Handedness, Birth Order and Homosexuality in Men'. In: *Laterality*, 13: 51–70.

49 Bos, H.W. & T.G.M. Sandfort (2010). 'Children's Gender Identity in Lesbian and Heterosexual Two-Parent Families'. In: *Sex Roles*, 62(1): 114–126.

50 Breedlove, S.M. (2017). 'Prenatal Influences on Human Sexual Orientation: Expectations versus Data'. In: *Arch Sex Behav*, Aug; 46(6): 1583–92.

51 Maccoby, E.E. et al. (1979). 'Concentrations of Sex Hormones in Umbilical-Cord Blood: Their Relation to Sex and Birth Order of Infants'. In: *Child Development*, Sept; 50(3): 632–42.

52 Blanchard, R. & A.F. Bogaert (1996). 'Homosexuality in Men and Number of Older Brothers'. In: *Am J Psychiatry*, 153: 27–31.

53 Blanchard, R. et al. (1997). 'H-Y Antigen and Homosexuality in Men'. In: *Journal of Theoretical Biology*, Apr 7; 185(3): 373–8.

### Chapter 5 – Old Choices in a New Paradise

1 Laar, A. van de (2014). *Onder het mes: de beroemdste patiënten en operaties uit de geschiedenis van de chirurgie*. Amsterdam: Thomas Rap.

2 https://www.pickle-publishing.com/papers/triple-crown-innocent-viii.htm

3 Reutrakul, S. & Van Cauter, E. (2018). 'Sleep influences on obesity, insulin resistance, and risk of type 2 diabetes'. In: *Metabolism*, July; 84: 56–66.

# Notes

4 Dickens, C. (2012). *The Pickwick Papers*. London: Penguin Classics.

5 Almuli, T. (2019). *Knap voor een dik meisje*. Amsterdam: Nijgh & Van Ditmar.

6 Hübel, C. et al. (2019). 'Epigenetics in eating disorders: a systematic review'. In: *Mol Psychiatry*, 24: 901–15.

7 Booij, L. & H. Steiger (2020). 'Applying epigenetic science to the understanding of eating disorders: a promising paradigm for research and practice'. In: *Curr Opin Psychiatry*, Nov; 33(6): 515–20.

8 http://psychclassics.yorku.ca/Pavlov/

9 Dimaline, R. et al. (2014). 'Novel roles of gastrin'. In: *J Physiol*, July 15; 592 (Pt 14): 2951–8.

10 Rehfeld, J.F. (2017). 'Cholecystokinin – From Local Gut Hormone to Ubiquitous Messenger'. In: *Front Endocrinol (Lausanne)*, 8: 47.

11 https://lion-nutrition.weebly.com/digestive-system.html

12 Broglio, F. et al. (2007). 'Brain-gut communication: cortistatin, somatostatin and ghrelin'. In: *Trends in Endocrinology & Metabolism*, Aug; 18(6): 246–51.

13 Cheng, H.L. et al. (2018). 'Ghrelin and Peptide YY Change During Puberty: Relationships with Adolescent Growth, Development, and Obesity'. In: *J Clin Endocrinol Metab*, Aug 1; 103(8): 2851–60.

14 Danziger, S., Levav, J. & L. Avnaim-Pesso (2011). 'Extraneous factors in judicial decisions'. In: *PNAS USA*, 108(17): 6889–92.

15 Linder, J.A. et al. (2014). 'Time of day and the decision to prescribe antibiotics'. In: *JAMA Intern Med*, 174(12): 2029–31.

16 Tal, A. et al. (2013). 'Fattening fasting: hungry grocery shoppers buy more calories, not more food'. In: *JAMA Intern Med*, 173(12): 1146–8.

17 https://books.google.be/books/about/De_borgelyke_tafel_om_lang_gesond_sonder.html?id=X4lbAAAAQAAJ&redir_esc=y

18 Walker, M. (2018). *Why We Sleep: The New Science of Sleep and Dreams*. New York: Scribner.

19 Ulhoa, M.A. (2015). 'Shift work and endocrine disorders'. In: *Int J Endocrinol*, 826249.

20 Mitler, M.M. et al. (1988). 'Catastrophes, sleep, and public policy: consensus report'. In: *Sleep*, 11(1): 100–9.

21 Leroyer, E. et al. (2014). 'Extended-duration hospital shifts, medical errors and patient mortality'. In: *Br J Hosp Med (Lond)*, 75(2): 96–101.

22 Ekirch, R. (2006). *Nacht en ontij. De geschiedenis van de nacht in de voorindustriële tijd*. Amsterdam: De Bezige Bij.

23 Mattingly, S.M. et al. (2021). 'The effects of seasons and weather on sleep patterns measured through longitudinal multimodal sensing'. In: *NPJ Digit Med*, Apr 28; 4(1): 76.

24  Yetish, G. et al. (2015). 'Natural sleep and its seasonal variations in three pre-industrial societies'. In: *Curr Biol*, Nov 2; 25(21): 2862–8.

25  Ekirch, R. (2002). *At Day's Close: A History of Nighttime*. London: Weidenfeld & Nicolson.

26  Wehr, T.A. (1992). 'In short photoperiods, human sleep is biphasic.' In: *J Sleep Res*, June; 1(2): 103–107.

27  Mesarwi, O. et al. (2013). 'Sleep disorders and the development of insulin resistance and obesity'. In: *Endocrinol Metab Clin North Am*, Sept; 42(3): 617–34.

28  Kojima, M. et al. (2013). 'Ghrelin discovery: a decade after'. In: *Endocr Dev*, 25: 1–4.

29  Anderberg, R.H. et al. (2016). 'The Stomach-Derived Hormone Ghrelin Increases Impulsive Behavior'. In: *Neuropsychopharmacology*, Apr; 41(5): 1199–209.

30  Parikh, S., Parikh, R., Michael, K. et al. (2022). 'Food-seeking behavior is triggered by skin ultraviolet exposure in males.' In: *Nat Metab*, 4: 883–900.

31  Theander, C. et al. (2006). 'Ghrelin action in the brain controls adipocyte metabolism'. In: *J Clin Invest*, July; 116(7): 1983–93.

32  King, W.C. et al. (2017). 'Alcohol and other substance use after bariatric surgery: prospective evidence from a U.S. multicenter cohort study'. In: *Surg Obes Relat Dis*, Aug; 13(8): 1392–402.

33  Hao, Z. et al. (2016). 'Does gastric bypass surgery change body weight set point?'. In: *Int J Obes Suppl*, Dec; 6 (Suppl 1): S37–S43.

34  Luchtman, D.W. et al. (2015). 'Defense of Elevated Body Weight Setpoint in Diet-Induced Obese Rats on Low Energy Diet Is Medicated by Loss of Melanocortin Sensitivity in the Paraventricular Hypothalmic Nucleus'. In: *PLoS One*, Oct 7; 10(10): e0139462.

35  Peters, A. et al. (2004). 'The selfish brain: competition for energy resources'. In: *Neurosci Biobehav Rev*, Apr; 28(2): 143–80.

36  Cummings, D.E. et al. (2002). 'Plasma ghrelin levels after diet-induced weight loss or gastric bypass surgery'. In: *N Engl J Med*, May 23; 346(21): 1623–30.

37  German, A.J. et al. (2006). 'The growing problem of obesity in dogs and cats'. In: *Journal of Nutrition*, July; 136(7): 1940S–1946S.

38  Ingalls, A.M. et al. (1950). 'Obese, a new mutation in the house mouse'. In: *J Hered*, Dec; 41(12): 3 17–8.

39  O'Rahilly, S. (2014). '20 years of leptin: what we know and what the future holds'. In: *J Endocrinol*, Oct; 223(1): E1–3.

40  Tausk, M. (1978). *Organon. De geschiedenis van een bijzondere Nederlanse onderneming*. Dekker & van de Vegt Nijmegen.

41  Goldschmidt, S. (2012). *De hormoonfabriek*. Amsterdam: Cossee.

42  Gershon, M. (1998). *The Second Brain*. USA: Harper.

43 Reiter, S. et al. (2017). 'On the Value of Reptilian Brains to Map the Evolution of the Hippocampal Formation'. In: *Brain Behav Evol*, 90(1): 41–52.
44 O'Neill, P.M. et al. (2018). 'Efficacy and safety of semaglutide compared with liraglutide and placebo for weight loss in patients with obesity: a randomised, double-blind, placebo and active controlled, dose-ranging, phase 2 trial'. In: *Lancet*, Aug 25; 392(10148): 637–49.
45 https://en.wikipedia.org/wiki/Natural_History_(Pliny)
46 See note 1.
47 https://en.wikipedia.org/wiki/Ivo_Pitanguy
48 https://medicine.uiowa.edu/surgery/content/memory-dr-edward-e-mason
49 Adams, T.D. et al. (2017). 'Weight and Metabolic Outcomes 12 Years after Gastric Bypass'. In: *N Engl J Med*, 377: 1143–55

## Chapter 6 – The Residents of Your Gut

1 Eiseman, B. et al. (1958). 'Fecal enema as an adjunct in the treatment of pseudomembranous enterocolitis'. In: *Surgery*, Nov; 44(5): 854–9.
2 Nood, E. van (2013). 'Duodenal infusion of donor feces for recurrent Clostridium difficile'. In: *NEJM*, 368(5): 407–15.
3 Enders, G. (2015). *Gut*. Scribe.
4 Knudsen, L.B. et al. (2019). 'The Discovery and Development of Liraglutide and Semaglutide'. In: *Front Endocrinol (Lausanne)*, Apr 12; 10: 155.
5 Covasa, M. et al. (2019). 'Intestinal Sensing by Gut Microbiota: Targeting Gut Peptides'. In: *Review Front Endocrinol (Lausanne)*, Feb 19; 10: 82.
6 Pijper, P. (2020). *Schatgravers en Scheppers*. Uitgeverij De Woordenwinkel, Zierikzee.
7 Engeland, C.G. et al. (2016). 'Psychological distress and salivary secretory immunity'. In: *Brain Behav Immun*, Feb; 52: 11–17.
8 Madsen, K.B. et al. (2013). 'Acute effects of continuous infusions of glucagon-like peptide (GLP)-1, GLP-2 and the combination (GLP-1+GLP-2) on intestinal absorption in short bowel syndrome (SBS) patients. A placebo-controlled study'. In: *Regul Pept*, June 10; 184: 30–9.
9 Fung, T.C et al. (2019). 'Intestinal serotonin and fluoxetine exposure modulate bacterial colonization in the gut'. In: *Nat Microbiol*, Dec; 4(12): 2064–73.
10 Kim, D.Y. et al. (2000). 'Serotonin: a mediator of the brain-gut connection'. In: *Am J Gastroenterol*, Oct; 95(10): 2698–709.
11 Neuman, H. et al. (2015). 'Microbial endocrinology: the

interplay between the microbiota and the endocrine system'. In: FEMS Microbiol Rev, July; 39(4): 509–21.

12 Gershon, M. (1999). *The Second Brain*. London: HarperCollins.

13 Fan, Y. et al. (2021). 'Gut microbiota in human metabolic health and disease'. In: *Nat Rev Microbiol*, Jan; 19(1): 55–71.

14 Bullmore, E. (2018). *Het ontstoken brein. Een radicaal nieuwe aanpak van depressie*. Amsterdam: Prometheus.

15 https://www.nobelprize.org/prizes/medicine/1958/lederberg/biographical/

16 Groot, P.F. de, et al. (2017). 'Fecal Microbiota Transplantation in Metabolic Syndrome: History, Present and Future'. In: *Gut Microbes*, May 4; 8(3): 253–67.

17 Koopman, N. et al. (2022). 'History of fecal transplantation; camel feces contains limited amounts of Bacillus subtilis spores and likely has no traditional role in the treatment of dysentery'. In: *PLoS One*, 17(8): e0272607.

18 Antonelli, G. et al. (2016). 'Evolution of the Koch postulates: towards a 21st-century understanding of microbial infection'. In: *Clin Microbiol Infect*, July; 22(7): 583–4.

19 Smits, L.P. et al. (2013). 'Therapeutic potential of fecal microbiota transplantation'. In: *Gastroenterology*, Nov; 145(5): 946–53.

20 Hanssen, N.M.J. et al. (2021). 'Fecal microbiota transplantation in human metabolic diseases: From a murky past to a bright future?'. In: *Cell Metab*, June 1; 33(6): 1098–1110.

21 Hartstra et al. (2020). 'Infusion of donor feces affects the gut-brain axis in humans with metabolic syndrome'. In: *Mol Metab*, Dec; 42: 101076.

22 Lyte, J.M. et al. (2020). 'Gut-brain axis serotonergic responses to acute stress exposure are microbiome-dependent'. In: *Neurogastroenterol Motil*, Nov; 32(11): e13881.

23 Meijnikman et al. (2022) 'Microbiome-derived ethanol in nonalcoholic fatty liver disease'. In: *Nature Medicine*, Oct; 28(10): 2100–6.

24 Chen, L. et al. (2021). 'Tryptophan-kynurenine metabolism: a link between the gut and brain for depression in inflammatory bowel disease'. In: *J Neuroinflammation*, 18: 135.

25 Esplugues, E. et al. (2011). 'Control of TH17 cells occurs in the small intestine'. In: *Nature*, July 28; 475(7357): 514–18.

26 Knezevic, J. et al. (2020). 'Thyroid-Gut-Axis: How Does the Microbiota Influence Thyroid Function?'. In: *Nutrients*, June; 12(6): 1769.

27 Heiss, C.N. et al. (2018). 'Gut Microbiota-Dependent Modulation of Energy Metabolism'. In: *J Innate Immun*, 10(3): 163–171.

28 Groot, P.F. de, et al. (2020). 'Donor metabolic characteristics drive effects of faecal microbiota transplantation on recipient

insulin sensitivity, energy expenditure and intestinal transit time'. In: *Gut*, Mar; 69(3): 502–12.

29  Chevalier, C. et al. (2015). 'Gut Microbiota Orchestrates Energy Homeostasis during Cold'. In: *Cell*, Dec 3; 163(6): 1360–74.

30  Smith, R.P. et al. (2019). 'Gut microbiome diversity is associated with sleep physiology in humans'. In: *PLoS One*, Oct 7; 14(10): e0222394.

31  Taiss, C.A. et al. (2014). 'Transkingdom control of microbiota diurnal oscillations promotes metabolic homeostasis'. In: *Cell*, Oct 23; 159(3): 514–29.

32  Kumar Dogra, S. et al. (2020). 'Gut Microbiota Resilience: Definition, Link to Health and Strategies for Intervention'. In: *Front Microbiol*, 11: 572921.

33  Garcia-Gutierrez, E. et al. (2019). 'Gut microbiota as a source of novel antimicrobials'. In: *Gut Microbes*, 10(1): 1–21.

34  Munger, E. et al. (2018). 'Reciprocal Interactions Between Gut Microbiota and Host Social Behavior'. In: *Front Integr Neurosci*, 12: 21.

35  Koren, O. et al. (2012). 'Host remodeling of the gut microbiome and metabolic changes during pregnancy'. In: *Cell*, Aug 3; 150(3): 470–80.

36  Fenneman A. (2023) 'A Comprehensive Review of Thyroid Hormone Metabolism in the Gut and Its Clinical Implications'. In: *Thyroid*, Jan; 33(1): 32–44.

37  Korpela, K. et al. (2020). 'Maternal Fecal Microbiota Transplantation in Cesarean-Born Infants Rapidly Restores Normal Gut Microbial Development: A Proof-of-Concept Study'. In: *Cell*, Oct 15; 183(2): 324–34.

38  Elsen, L.W.J. van den, et al. (2019). 'Shaping the Gut Microbiota by Breastfeeding: The Gateway to Allergy Prevention?'. In: *Front Pediatr*, 7: 47.

39  Song, S.J. et al. (2013). 'Cohabiting family members share microbiota with one another and with their dogs'. In: *eLife*, Apr 16; 2: e00458.

40  Costea, P.I. et al. (2018). 'Enterotypes in the landscape of gut microbial community composition'. In: *Nat Microbiol*, Jan; 3(1): 8–16.

41  Yao, Z. et al. (2020). 'Relation of Gut Microbes and L-Thyroxine Through Altered Thyroxine Metabolism in Subclinical Hypothyroidism Subjects'. In: Front Cell Infect Microbiol, 10: 495.

42  Krogh Pedersen, H. et al. (2016). 'Human gut microbes impact host serum metabolome and insulin sensitivity'. In: *Nature*, July 21; 535(7612): 376–81.

43  Blaser, M. (2015). *Missing Microbes: How Killing Bacteria Creates Modern Plagues*. London: Oneworld Publications.

44 Clemente, J.C. et al. (2015). 'The microbiome of uncontacted Amerindians'. In: *Sci Adv*, Apr 3; 1(3): e1500183.
45 Blaser, M. (2015). *Missing Microbes: How Killing Bacteria Creates Modern Plagues*. London: Oneworld Publications.
46 https://taymount.com
47 Niazi, A.K. et al. (2011). 'Thyroidology over the ages'. In: *Indian J Endocrinol Metab*, July; 15(Suppl2): S121–6.

## Chapter 7 – Hormones Make or Break the Man and Woman

1 Golden, S.H. et al. (2009). 'Clinical review: Prevalence and incidence of endocrine and metabolic disorders in the United States: a comprehensive review'. In: *J Clin Endocrinol Metab*, June 1; 94(6): 1853–78.
2 Mantel, H. (2016). *De geest geven*. Translated by Gerda G. Baardman and Anne Jongeling. Amsterdam: AtlasContact.
3 Djerassi, C. (2001). *This Man's Pill: Reflections on the 50th Birthday of the Pill*. Oxford: Oxford University Press.
4 Rosing, J., Middeldorp, S. et al. (1999). 'Low-dose oral contraceptives and acquired resistance to activated protein C: a randomised cross-over study'. In: *Lancet*, Dec 11; 354(9195): 2036–40.
5 Pletzer, B.A. & H.H. Kerschbaum (2014). '50 years of hormonal contraception –time to find out, what it does to our brain'. In: *Front Neurosci*, Aug 21; 8: 256.
6 Schaffir, J. et al. (2016). 'Combined hormonal contraception and its effects on mood: a critical review'. In: *Eur J Contracept Reprod Health Care*, Oct; 21(5): 347–55.
7 Skovlund, C.W. et al. (2018). 'Association of Hormonal Contraception with Suicide Attempts and Suicides'. In: *Am J Psychiatry*, Apr 1; 175(4): 336–42.
8 Zimmerman, Y. et al. (2014). 'The effect of combined oral contraception on testosterone levels in healthy women: a systematic review and meta-analysis'. In: *Hum Reprod Update*, Jan; 20(1): 76–105.
9 Panzer, C. et al. (2006). 'Impact of oral contraceptives on sex hormone-binding globulin and androgen levels: a retrospective study in women with sexual dysfunction'. In: *J Sex Med*, 2006 Jan; 3(1): 104–13.
10 Nielsen, S.E. et al. (2011). 'Hormonal contraception usage is associated with altered memory for an emotional story'. In: *Neurobiol Learn Mem*, Sept; 96(2): 378–84.
11 Mordecai, K.L. et al. (2017). 'Cortisol reactivity and emotional memory after psychosocial stress in oral contraceptive users'. In: *J Neurosci Res*, Jan 2; 95(1–2): 126–35.
12 Toni, R. (2000). 'Ancient views on the

hypothalamic-pituitary-thyroid axis: an historical and epistemological perspective'. In: *Pituitary*, Oct; 3(2): 83–95.

13 Janicki-Deverts, D. et al. 'Basal salivary cortisol secretion and susceptibility to upper respiratory infection'. In: *Brain Behav Immun*, Mar; 53: 255–61.

14 Fröhlich, E. et al. (2017). 'Thyroid Autoimmunity: Role of Anti-thyroid Antibodies in Thyroid and Extra-Thyroidal Diseases'. In: *Front Immunol*, 8: 521.

15 https://endodc.com/news/thyroid-conditions-and-digestive-problems#:~:text=Hypothyroidism%2C%20or%20too%20little%20thyroid,constipation%2C%20forgetfulness%20and%20weight%20gain

16 Chaker, L. et al. (2017). 'Hypothyroidism'. In: *Lancet*, Sept 23; 390(10101): 1550–62.

17 Martino, E. (2012). 'Endocrinology and Art. Madonna del Rosario (Lady of the rosary) – Michelangelo Merisi called Caravaggio (1571–1610)'. In: *Journal of Endocrinological Investigation*, 35(2): 243.

18 Papapetrou, P.D. (2015). 'The philosopher Socrates had exophthalmos (a term coined by Plato) and probably Graves' disease'. In: *Hormones (Athens)*, Jan–Mar; 14(1): 167–71.

19 https://thyroidwellness.com/blogs/default-blog/president-bush-s-graves-disease-story-and-the-potential-triggers-of-his-thyroid-condition

20 https://columbiasurgery.org/news/2015/09/03/history-medicine-leonardo-da-vinci-and-elusive-thyroid-0

21 Laios, K. et al. (2019). 'From thyroid cartilage to thyroid gland'. In: *Folia Morphol*, 78(1): 171–3.

22 Niazi, A.K. et al. (2011). 'Thyroidology over the ages'. In: *Indian J Endocrinol Metab*, July; 15(Suppl2): S121–S126.

23 Ibid.

24 Leung, A.M. et al. (2012). 'History of U.S. iodine fortification and supplementation'. In: *Nutrients*, Nov; 4(11): 1740–46.

25 Meijer van Putten, J.B. (1997). 'Jodiumtekort'. In: *Ned Tijdschr Geneeskd*, 141:453–4.

26 Loos, V. (2008). 'A thyrotoxicosis outbreak due to dietary pills in Paris'. In: *Ther Clin Risk Manag*, Dec; 4(6): 1375–9.

27 Parmar, M. et al. (2003). 'Recurrent hamburger thyrotoxicosis'. In: *CMAJ*, Sept 2; 169(5): 415–17.

28 Ranabir, S. et al. (2011). 'Stress and hormones'. In *Indian J Endocrinol Metab*, Jan–Mar; 15(1): 18–22.

29 Bérard, L. (1916). 'La maladie de Basedow et la guerre'. In: *Bull Acad. de méd*, 76: 428.

30 Weisschedel-Freiburg, E. (1953). 'Characteristics of Basedow's disease and hyperthyreoses after the war; therapy with radioiodine'. In: *Langenbecks Arch. u. Dtsch. Z. Clair*, 273: 817–19.

31 Paunkovic, N. et al. (1998). 'The significant increase in

incidence of Graves' disease in eastern Serbia during the civil war in the former Yugoslavia (1992 to 1995)'. In: *Thyroid*, Jan; 8(1): 37–41.

32 https://www.brainimmune.com/caleb-parry-and-the-relationship-between-hyperthyroidism-and-stress/

33 https://www.schilddruesengesellschaft.at/sites/osdg.at/fles/upload/15%20Weissel%20-%20Schilddruese%20und%20Stressful%20Life%20Events.pdf

34 Vita, R. et al. (2009). 'A patient with stress-related onset and exacerbations of Graves disease'. In: *Nat Clin Pract Endocrinol Metab*, Jan; 5(1): 55–61.

35 https://www.thyroid.org/thyroid-disease-pregnancy/

36 Michels, A.W. et al. (2010). 'Immunologic endocrine disorders'. In: *J Allergy Clin Immunol*, Feb; 125(2 Suppl 2): S226–S237.

37 https://neuroendoimmune.wordpress.com/2013/04/16/horror-autotoxicus-the-story-of-autoimmunity/

38 Ngo, S.T. et al. (2014). 'Gender differences in autoimmune disease'. In: *Frontiers in Neuroendocrinology*, 35(3): 347–69.

39 Quintero, O. et al. (2012). 'Autoimmune disease and gender: plausible mechanisms for the female predominance of autoimmunity'. In: *J Autoimmun*, May; 38(2-3): J109–19.

40 Flak, M.B. et al. (2013). 'Immunology. Welcome to the microgenderome'. In: *Science*, Mar 1; 339(6123): 1044–5.

41 Fuhri Snethlage, C.M. et al. (2021). 'Auto-immunity and the gut microbiome in type 1 diabetes: Lessons from rodent and human studies'. In: *Best Pract Res Clin Endocrinol Metab*, May; 35(3): 101544.

42 http://www.endocrinesurgery.net.au/adrenal-history/

43 Owen, D. (2008). *Zieke wereldleiders. Hoe overmoed, depressie en andere aandoeningen politieke beslissingen sturen*. Amsterdam: Nieuw Amsterdam.

44 Horby, P. et al. (2021). 'Dexamethasone in Hospitalized Patients with Covid-19'. In: *N Engl J Med*, Feb 25; 384(8): 693–704.

45 Lee, D. et al. (2015). 'Technical and clinical aspects of cortisol as a biochemical marker of chronic stress'. In: *BMB Rep*, Apr; 48(4): 209–16.

46 https://www.historynet.com/jack-kennedy-dr-feelgood.htm

47 http://www.history.com/topics/us-presidents/kennedy-nixon-debates

48 Mandel, L.R. (2009). 'Endocrine and autoimmune aspects of the health history of John F. Kennedy'. In: *Ann Intern Med*, Sept 1; 151(5): 350–4.

49 Carney, J.A. (1995). 'The Search for Harvey Cushing's Patient, Minnie G., and the Cause of Her Hypercortisolism'. In: *Am J Surg Path*, 19(1): 100–8.

50 Lupien, S. (2014). *Well Stressed: Manage Stress Before It Turns Toxic*. HarperCollins Canada.

51  https://www.nobelprize.org/prizes/medicine/1950/hench/facts/
52  Owen L.D. (2005). 'The effect of Prime Minister Anthony Eden's illness on his decision-making during the Suez crisis'. In: *QJM*, June; 98(6): 387–402.
53  Hinz, L. et al. (2011). 'Why did Harvey Cushing misdiagnose Cushing's disease? The enigma of endocrinological diagnoses'. In: *UWOMJ*, 79(1): 43–6.
54  Househam, A.M. et al. (2017). 'The Effects of Stress and Meditation on the Immune System, Human Microbiota, and Epigenetics'. In: *Adv Mind Body Med*, Fall; 31(4): 10–25.
55  Keown, D. (2014). *The Spark in the Machine*. Jessica Kingsley Publishers.
56  Ma, X. (2017). 'The Effect of Diaphragmatic Breathing on Attention, Negative Affect and Stress in Healthy Adults'. In: *Front Psychol*, 8; 874.
57  Benvenutti, M.J. et al. (2017). 'A single session of hatha yoga improves stress reactivity and recovery after an acute psychological stress task – A counterbalanced, randomized-crossover trial in healthy individuals'. In: *Complement Ther Med*, Dec; 35: 120–6.
58  Thind, H. et al. (2017). 'The effects of yoga among adults with type 2 diabetes: A systematic review and meta-analysis'. In: *Prev Med*, Dec; 105: 116–26.
59  Nilakanthan, S. et al. (2016). 'Effect of 6 months intense Yoga practice on lipid profile, thyroxine medication and serum TSH level in women suffering from hypothyroidism: A pilot study'. In: *J Complement Integr Med*, June 1; 13(2): 189–93.
60  Chu, P. et al. (2016). 'The effectiveness of yoga in modifying risk factors for cardiovascular disease and metabolic syndrome: A systematic review and meta-analysis of randomized controlled trials'. In: *European Journal of Preventive Cardiology*, 23(3), 291–307.
61  Lequin, R.M. et al. (2002). 'Marius Tausk (1902–1990), influential endocrinologist and producer of medicines; a retrospect to mark the centenary of his birth'. In: *Ned Tijdschr Geneeskd*, Feb 16; 146(7): 327–30.
62  Knegtmans, P.J. (2014). *Geld, ijdelheid en hormonen. Ernst Lacqueur (1880-1947), hoogleraar en ondernemer*. Amsterdam: Boom.
63  https://www.nobelprize.org/prizes/chemistry/1939/butenandt/biographical/
64  Anonymous (1896). 'The Brown Séquard method of testicular extract therapy'. In: *JAMA*, 26(10): 488.
65  https://historianet.nl/oorlog/tweede-wereldoorlog/hitler/hitler-was-in-de-tweede-wereldoorlog-aan-de-drugs
66  Williams, B.R. et al. (2017). 'Hormone Replacement: The Fountain of Youth?'. In: *Prim Care*, Sept; 44(3): 481–98.
67  Wade, N. (1972). 'Anabolic Steroids: Doctors Denounce Them,

but Athletes Aren't Listening'. In: *Science*, June 30; 176(4042): 1399–403.
68  Nieschlag, E. & E. Voron (2015). 'Mechanisms in Endocrinology: Medical consequences of doping with anabolic androgenic steroids: effects on reproductive functions'. In: *Eur J Endocrinol*, Aug; 173(2): R47–58.
69  Tod, D. et al. (2016). 'Muscle dysmorphia: current insights'. In: *Psychol Res Behav Manag*, 9: 179–188.
70  https://wgs160.wordpress.com/2014/10/13/the-evolution-of-gi-joe/
71  Herman, C.W. et al. (2014). 'The very high premature mortality rate among active professional wrestlers is primarily due to cardiovascular disease'. In: *PLoS One*, Nov; 9(11): e109945.
72  Achar, S. et al. (2010). 'Cardiac and metabolic effects of anabolic-androgenic steroid abuse on lipids, blood pressure, left ventricular dimensions, and rhythm'. In: *American Journal of Cardiology*, Sept; 106(6): 893–901.
73  https://www.fda.gov/consumers/consumer-updates/teens-and-steroids-dangerous-combo
74  http://www.europarl.europa.eu/news/en/press-room/20120314ipr40752/win-win-ending-to-the-hormone-beef-trade-war

## Chapter 8 – The Change

1  Lobo, R. (2003). 'Early ovarian ageing: a hypothesis. What is early ovarian ageing?'. In: *Hum Reprod*, Sept; 18(9): 1762–4.
2  Buckler H. (2005). 'The menopause transition: endocrine changes and clinical symptoms'. In: *J Br Menopause Soc*, June; 11(2): 61–5.
3  Greenblatt, R.B. et al. (1976). 'Estrogen-androgen levels in aging men and women: therapeutic considerations'. In: *J Am Geriatr Soc*, Apr; 24(4): 173–8.
4  Alpanes, M. et al. (2012). 'Management of postmenopausal virilization'. In: *Journal of Clinical Endocrinology & Metabolism*, 97 (8): 2584–8.
5  Aristotle edited by Ogle, W. (2010). *De partibus animalium*. Bibliolife, USA.
6  https://en.wikipedia.org/wiki/Trotula
7  Muscat Baron, Y. (2012). *A History of the Menopause*. Department of Obstetrics and Gynaecology, Faculty of Medicine & Surgery, University of Malta.
8  https://en.wikipedia.org/wiki/Climacteric_year
9  https://www.laphamsquarterly.org/roundtable/signifcant-life-event
10  Livesley, B. (1977). 'The climacteric disease'. In: J Am Geriatr Soc, Apr; 25(4): 162–6.

# Notes

11  Rees, M. et al. (2021). 'Global consensus recommendations on menopause in the workplace: A European Menopause and Andropause Society (EMAS) position statement'. In: *Maturitas*, Sept; 151: 55–62.

12  https://www.nrc.nl/nieuws/2011/01/08/de-overgang-is-de-weg-naar-de-dood-11986165-a21417

13  Ayranci, U. et al. (2010). 'Menopause status and attitudes in a Turkish midlife female population: an epidemiological study'. In: *BMC Womens Health*, Jan 11; 10: 1.

14  Jones, E.K. et al. (2012). 'Menopause and the influence of culture: another gap for Indigenous Australian women?'. In: *BMC Womens Health*, 12: 43.

15  Flint, M. (1975). 'The menopause: reward or punishment?'. In: *Psychosomatics*, 16: 161–3.

16  Hoga, L. et al. (2015). 'Women's experience of menopause: a systematic review of qualitative evidence'. In: *JBI Database System Rev Implement Rep*, Sept 16; 13(8): 250–337.

17  Beyene, Y. (1986). 'Cultural significance and physiological manifestations of menopause. A biocultural analysis'. In: *Cult Med Psychiatry*, Mar; 10(1): 47–71.

18  Mar, S.O. (2020). 'Rural-urban difference in natural menopausal age'. In: *International Journal of Women's Health and Reproduction Sciences*, 8(2): 112–18.

19  Peccei, J.S. (1995). 'A hypothesis for the origin and evolution of menopause'. In: *Maturitas*, Feb; 21(2): 83–9.

20  Kuhle, B.X. (2007). 'An evolutionary perspective on the origin and ontogeny of menopause'. In: *Maturitas*, Aug 20; 57(4): 329–37.

21  Ellis, S. et al. (2018). 'Postreproductive lifespans are rare in mammals'. In: *Ecol Evol*, Jan 31; 8(5): 2482–94.

22  Stockwell, S. (1983). 'Classics in oncology. George Tomas Beatson, M.D. (1848-1933)'. In: *Cancer J Clin*, Mar–Apr; 33(2): 105–21.

23  https://www.nobelprize.org/prizes/medicine/1966/huggins/facts/

24  Wilson, R.A. (1966). *Feminine Forever*. New York: Evans.

25  Chung, H.F. et al. (2021). 'Age at menarche and risk of vasomotor menopausal symptoms: a pooled analysis of six studies'. In: *BJOG*, Feb; 128(3): 603–13.

26  Saccomani, S. et al. 'Does obesity increase the risk of hot flashes among midlife women?: A population-based study'. In: *Menopause*, Sep; 24(9): 1065–70.

27  Ameye, L. et al. (2014). 'Menopausal hormone therapy use in 17 European countries during the last decade'. In: *Maturitas*, Nov; 79(3): 287–91.

28  Rossouw, J.E. et al. (2002). 'Risks and benefits of estrogen plus progestin in healthy postmenopausal women: principal results from the Women's Health Initiative randomized controlled trial'. In: *JAMA*, July 17; 288(3): 321–33.

29  Beral V. et al (2015). 'Menopausal hormone use and ovarian cancer risk: individual participant meta-analysis of 52 epidemiological studies'. In: *Lancet*, May 9; 385(9980): 1835–42.

30  Chen, M.N. et al. (2015). 'Efficacy of phytoestrogens for menopausal symptoms: a meta-analysis and systematic review'. In: *Climacteric*, Mar; 18(2): 260–9.

31  Spalek, K. et al. (2019). 'Women using hormonal contraceptives show increased valence ratings and memory performance for emotional information'. In: *Neuropsychopharmacology*, 44(7): 1258–64.

32  Weber, M.T. et al. (2014). 'Cognition and mood in perimenopause: a systematic review and meta-analysis'. In: *J Steroid Biochem Mol Biol*, July; 142: 90–8.

33  Caldwell, B.M. et al. (1954). 'An evaluation of sex hormone replacement in aged women'. In: *J Genet Psychol*, Dec; 85(2): 181–200.

34  Berg, J.S. et al. (2000). 'Early menopause presenting with mood symptoms in a student aviator'. In: *Aviat Space Environ Med*, Mar; 71(3): 251–4.

35  Henderson, V.W. (2011). 'Gonadal hormones and cognitive aging: a midlife perspective'. In: *Womens Health (Lond Engl)*, Jan; 7(1): 81–93.

36  Luine, V.N. (2014). 'Estradiol and cognitive function: past, present and future'. In: *Horm Behav*, Sept; 66(4): 602–18.

37  https://en.wikipedia.org/wiki/Jubilee_(biblical)

38  Ginsberg, J. (1991). 'What determines the age at the menopause?'. In: *BMJ*, June 1; 302(6788): 1288–9.

39  Haller-Kikkatalo, K. et al. (2015). 'The prevalence and phenotypic characteristics of spontaneous premature ovarian failure: a general population registry-based study'. In: *Human Reproduction*, May; 30(5): 1229–38.

40  http://www.dailymail.co.uk/femail/article-2125245/I-went-menopause-Hot-flushes-classroom-Hrt-shed-kiss-Knowing-d-baby-But-shocking-Amanda-s-ordeal-far-unique.html

41  Bentzen, J.G. et al. (2013). 'Maternal menopause as a predictor of anti-Mullerian hormone level and antral follicle count in daughters during reproductive age'. In: *Hum Reprod*, Jan; 28(1): 247–55.

42  Evans, D.G. et al. (2014). 'The Angelina Jolie effect: how high celebrity profile can have a major impact on provision of cancer related services'. In: *Breast Cancer Res*, Sept 19; 16(5): 442.

43  Depmann, M. et al. (2016). 'Can we predict age at natural menopause using ovarian reserve tests or mother's age at menopause? A systematic literature review'. In: *Menopause*, Feb; 23(2): 224–32.

44  Murabito, J.M. et al. (2005). 'Heritability of age at natural

menopause in the Framingham Heart Study'. In: *J Clin Endocrinol Metab*, June; 90(6): 3427–30.

45 Snieder, H. et al. (1998). 'Genes control the cessation of a woman's reproductive life: a twin study of hysterectomy and age at menopause'. In: *J Clin Endocrinol Metab*, June; 83(6): 1875–80.

46 Schmidt, C.W. (2017). 'Age at Menopause: Do Chemical Exposures Play a Role?'. In: *Environ Health Perspect*, June; 125(6): 062001.

47 https://en.wikipedia.org/wiki/Seveso_disaster

48 Eskenazi, B. et al. (2005). 'Serum dioxin concentrations and age at menopause'. In: *Environ Health Perspect*, July; 113(7): 858–62.

49 Ding, N. (2020). 'Associations of Perfluoroalkyl Substances with Incident Natural Menopause: The Study of Women's Health Across the Nation'. In: *J Clin Endocrinol Metab*, 105(9): e3169–82.

50 Coperchini, F. (2020). 'Thyroid Disrupting Effects of Old and New Generation PFAS'. In: *Front Endocrinol (Lausanne)*, 11: 612320.

51 Chevrier, J. (2014). 'Serum dioxin concentrations and thyroid hormone levels in the Seveso Women's Health Study'. In: *Am J Epidemiol*, Sept 1; 180(5): 490–8.

52 Chow, E.T. et al. (2016). 'Cosmetics use and age at menopause: is there a connection?'. In: *Fertil Steril*, Sept 15; 106(4): 978–90.

53 Bonneux, L. et al. (2008). 'Sensible family planning: do not have children too late, but not too early either'. In: *Ned Tijdschr Geneeskd*, 152: 1507–12.

54 Wang, J. et al. (2006). 'In vitro fertilization (IVF): a review of 3 decades of clinical innovation and technological advancement'. In: *Ter Clin Risk Manag*, Dec; 2(4): 355–64.

55 Kawamura, K. et al. (2016). 'Activation of dormant follicles: a new treatment for premature ovarian failure?'. In: *Curr Opin Obstet Gynecol*, June; 28(3): 217–22.

56 Zhang, L. et al. (2021). 'Autotransplantation of the ovarian cortex after invitro activation for infertility treatment: a shortened procedure'. In: *Human Reproduction*, Aug; 36(8): 2134–47.

57 Farquhar, C. et al. (2013). 'Assisted reproductive technology: an overview of Cochrane Reviews'. In: *Cochrane Database Syst Rev*, Aug 22; (8): CD010537.

58 https://www.nytimes.com/1984/04/11/us/first-baby-born-of-frozen-embryo.html

59 See note 52.

60 http://www.businessinsider.com/egg-freezing-at-facebook-apple-google-hot-new-perk-2017-9

61 https://www.theatlantic.com/technology/archive/2012/06/the-ivf-panic-all-hell-will-break-loose-politically-and-morally-all-over-the-world/258954/

62 https://www.nvog.nl/wp-content/uploads/2017/12/Anovulatie-en-kinderwens-2.0-12-11-2004.pdf
63 Sandin, S. et al. (2013). 'Autism and mental retardation among offspring born after in vitro fertilization'. In: *JAMA*, July 3; 310(1): 75–84.
64 Zhu, J.L. et al. (2009). 'Parental infertility and sexual maturation in children'. In: *Hum Reprod*, Feb; 24(2): 445–50.
65 Lyngsø, J. et al. (2019). 'Impact of female daily coffee consumption on successful fertility treatment: a Danish cohort study'. In: *Fertil Steril*, July; 112(1): 120–9.
66 https://www.huffingtonpost.co.uk/2015/01/19/worlds-oldest-mother-omkali-singh_n_6501268.html
67 https://www.timesnownews.com/health/article/meet-tiantian-the-baby-boy-who-was-born-four-years-after-his-parents-died-in-a-car-crash-in-china/216924
68 http://www.bbc.com/news/world-asia-china-43724395
69 https://www.independent.co.uk/life-style/health-and-families/embryo-24-years-frozen-born-baby-longest-ever-tina-benjamin-gibson-emma-wren-nedc-tennessee-a8119776.html
70 (see note 10)
71 Bribiescas, R. (2016). *How Men Age*. USA: Princeton University Press.
72 Karasik, D. et al. (2005). 'Disentangling the genetic determinants of human aging: biological age as an alternative to the use of survival measures'. In: *J Gerontol A Biol Sci Med Sci*, May; 60(5): 574–87.
73 Wu, F.C.W. et al. (2008). 'Hypothalamic-pituitary-testicular axis disruptions in older men are differentially linked to age and modifiable risk factors: the European Male Aging Study'. In: *J Clin Endocrinol Metab*, 93(7): 2737.
74 Amore, M. et al. (2012). 'Partial androgen deficiency, depression, and testosterone supplementation in aging men'. In: *Int J Endocrinol*, 2012: 280724.
75 Wolffers, I. (2006). *Heimwee naar de lust. Over seks en ziekte.* Amsterdam: Contact.
76 Jones, G.H. et al. (2015). 'Traumatic andropause after combat injury'. In: *BMJ Case Rep*, 2015: bcr2014207924.
77 Tajar, A. et al. (2012). 'Characteristics of androgen deficiency in late-onset hypogonadism: results from the European Male Aging Study (EMAS)'. In: *J Clin Endocrinol Metab*, May; 97(5): 1508–16.
78 Snyder, P.J., Bauer, D.C., Ellenberg, S.S. et al. (2024). *New England Journal of Medicine*, 390(3): 203–11.
79 De Kruif, P. (1945). *The Male Hormone*. New York: Harcourt, Brace and Company.
80 https://lowtcenter.com

80 Bachmann, E. et al. (2014). 'Testosterone induces erythrocytosis via increased erythropoietin and suppressed hepcidin: evidence for a new erythropoietin/hemoglobin set point'. In: *J Gerontol A Biol Sci Med Sci*, June; 69(6): 725–35.

82 Nieschlag, E. et al. (2014). 'Testosterone deficiency: a historical perspective'. In: *Asian J Androl*, Mar–Apr; 16(2): 161–8.

83 Herman, C.W. et al. (2014). 'The very high premature mortality rate among active professional wrestlers is primarily due to cardiovascular disease'. In: *PLoS One*, Nov; 9(11): e109945.

84 Achar, S. et al. (2010). 'Cardiac and metabolic effects of anabolic-androgenic steroid abuse on lipids, blood pressure, left ventricular dimensions, and rhythm'. In: *American Journal of Cardiology*, Sept; 106(6): 893–901.

85 Gentil, P. et al. (2017). 'Nutrition, Pharmacological and Training Strategies Adopted by Six Bodybuilders: Case Report and Critical Review'. In: *Eur J Transl Myol*, Feb 24; 27(1): 6247.

86 Kelly, D.M. et al. (2015). 'Testosterone and obesity'. In: *Obes Rev*, July; 16(7): 581–606.

87 Smith, G. et al. (2004). 'Treatments of homosexuality in Britain since the 1950s – an oral history: the experience of patients'. In: *BMJ*, Feb 21; 328(7437): 427.

## Chapter 9 – A New Balance

1 Gray, J. (1992). *Men Are from Mars, Women are from Venus*. New York: HarperCollins.

2 Karastergiou, K. et al. (2012). 'Sex differences in human adipose tissues – the biology of pear shape'. In: *Biol Sex Differ*, 3: 13.

3 Tomassoni, D. et al. (2014). 'Gender and age related differences in foot morphology'. In: *Maturitas*, Dec; 79(4): 421–7.

4 Sforza, C. et al. (2008). 'Spontaneous blinking in healthy persons: an optoelectronic study of eyelid motion'. In: *Ophthalmic Physiol Opt*, July; 28(4): 345–53.

5 https://www.nytimes.com/2020/04/27/well/live/car-accidents-deaths-men-women.html

6 Pataky, M.W. et al. (2021). 'Hormonal and Metabolic Changes of Aging and the Influence of Lifestyle Modifications'. In: , Mar; 96(3): 788–814.

7 Ali, L. et al. (2011). 'Physiological changes in scalp, facial and body hair after the menopause: a cross-sectional population-based study of subjective changes'. In: *Br J Dermatol*, Mar; 164(3): 508–13.

8 https://en.wikipedia.org/wiki/Wilgefortis

9 New, M.I. (1993). 'Pope Joan: a recognizable syndrome'. In: *Clin Endocrinol Metab*, Jan; 76(1): 3–13.

10 https://www.nomadbarber.com/blogs/barbering/masai-male-grooming
11 https://www.telegraph.co.uk/health-fitness/body/finasteride-does-donald-trumps-favourite-hair-loss-treatment/
12 Gunn, D.A. et al. (2009). 'Why some women look young for their age'. In: *PLoS One*, Dec 1; 4(12): e8021.
13 Mandal, S. et al. (2017). 'Automated Age Prediction Using Wrinkles Features of Facial Images and Neural Network'. In: *International Journal of Emerging Engineering Research and Technology*, Feb; 5(2): 12–20.
14 Stevenson, S., Thornton, J. (2007). 'Effect of estrogens on skin aging and the potential role of SERMS'. In: *Clin Interv Aging*, Sept; 2(3): 283–97.
15 Thornton, M.J. (2013). 'Estrogens and aging skin'. In: *Dermatoendocrinol*, Apr 1; 5(2): 264–70.
16 Vermeulen, A. et al. (2002). 'Estradiol in elderly men'. In: *Aging Male*, June; 5(2): 98–102.
17 Mydlova, M. et al. (2015). 'Sexual dimorphism of facial appearance in ageing human adults: A cross-sectional study'. In: *Forensic Sci Int*, Dec; 257: 519.
18 Verdonck, A. et al. (1999). 'Effect of low-dose testosterone treatment on craniofacial growth in boys with delayed puberty'. In: *Eur J Orthod*, Apr; 21(2): 137–43.
19 Teede, H.J. et al. (2018). 'Recommendations from the international evidence-based guideline for the assessment and management of polycystic ovary syndrome'. In: *Clin Endocrinol (Oxf)*, Sept; 89(3): 251–68.
20 Urban, J.E. et al. (2016). 'Evaluation of morphological changes in the adult skull with age and sex'. In: *J Anat*, Dec; 229(6): 838–46.
21 Robertson, J.M. et al. (2017). 'Sexually Dimorphic Faciometrics in Humans From Early Adulthood to Late Middle Age: Dynamic, Declining, and Differentiated'. In: *Evol Psychol*, July–Sept; 15(3): 1474704917730640.
22 Zube, M. (1982). 'Changing Behavior and Outlook of Aging Men and Women: Implications for Marriage in the Middle and Later Years'. In: *Family Relations*, Jan; 31(1): 147–56.
23 http://www.psychiatrictimes.com/geriatric-psychiatry/geriatric-depression-does-gender-make-difference
24 Coren, S. et al. (1999). 'Sex differences in elderly suicide rates: Some predictive factors'. In: *Aging & Mental Health*, 3(2): 112–8.
25 Hahn, T. et al. (2017). 'Facial width-to-height ratio differs by social rank across organizations, countries, and value systems'. In: *PLoS One*, Nov 9; 12(11): e0187957.
26 Re, D.E. et al. (2013). 'Looking like a leader – facial shape predicts perceived height and leadership ability'. In: *PLoS One*, 8(12): e80957.

# Notes

27  Antonaik, J. et al. (2009). 'Predicting elections: child's play!'. In: *Science*, Feb 27; 323(5918): 1183.
28  Overbeek, B. (2016). *Mannen en/of Vrouwen*. Veghel: Libris.
29  Morrison, M.D. et al. (1986). 'Voice disorders in the elderly'. In: *J Otolaryngol*, Aug; 15(4): 231–4.
30  https://www.webmd.com/menopause/news/20040316/voice-change-is-overlooked-menopause-symptom#2
31  Pavela Banai, L. (2017). 'Voice in different phases of menstrual cycle among naturally cycling women and users of hormonal contraceptives'. In: *PLoS One*, 12(8): e0183462.
32  Puts, D.A. (2005). 'Mating context and menstrual phase affect women's preferences for male voice pitch'. In: *Evolution and Human Behavior*, Sept; 26(5): 388–97.
33  Schild, C. et al. (2020). 'Linking human male vocal parameters to perceptions, body morphology, strength and hormonal profiles in contexts of sexual selection'. In: *Sci Rep*, Dec 4; 10(1): 21296.
34  Aung, T. et al. (2020). 'Voice pitch: a window into the communication of social power'. In: *Curr Opin Psychol*, June; 33: 154–61.
35  Mody, L. et al. (2014). 'Urinary tract infections in older women: a clinical review'. In: *JAMA*, Feb 26; 311(8): 844–54.
36  Jung, J. et al. (2012). 'Clinical and functional anatomy of the urethral sphincter'. In: *Int Neurourol J*, Sept; 16(3): 102–6.
37  Heidari, B. (2011). 'Knee osteoarthritis prevalence, risk factors, pathogenesis and features: Part I'. In: *Caspian J Intern Med*, Spring; 2(2): 205–12.
38  Souza, A.A. et al. (2013). 'Association between knee alignment, body mass index and physical fitness variables among students: a cross-sectional study'. In: *Rev Bras Ortop*, June 11; 48(1): 46–51.
39  Milic, J. et al. (2018). 'Menopause, ageing, and alcohol use disorders in women'. In: *Maturitas*, May; 111: 100–9.
40  Devries, M.C. et al. (2006). 'Menstrual cycle phase and sex influence muscle glycogen utilization and glucose turnover during moderate-intensity endurance exercise'. In: *Am J Physiol Regul Integr Comp Physiol*, Oct; 291(4): R1120-8.
41  Carter, S.L. et al. (2001). 'Substrate utilization during endurance exercise in men and women after endurance training'. In: *Am J Physiol Endocrinol Metab*, June; 280(6): E898–907.
42  https://www.hartstichting.nl/hart-en-vaatziekten/vrouwen-en-hart-en-vaatziekten
43  Mehta, L. (2016). 'Acute Myocardial Infarction in Women: A Scientific Statement from the American Heart Association'. In: *Circulation*, 133(9): 916–47.
44  Wittekoek, J. (2017). *Het vrouwenhart*. Hilversum: Lucht.
45  Lansky, A.J. et al. (2012). 'Gender and the extent of coronary

atherosclerosis, plaque composition, and clinical outcomes in acute coronary syndromes'. In: *JACC Cardiovasc Imaging*, Mar; 5(3 Suppl): S62–72.

46 Grundtvig, M. et al. (2009). 'Sex-based differences in premature first myocardial infarction caused by smoking: twice as many years lost by women as by men'. In: *Eur J Cardiovasc Prev Rehabil*, Apr; 16(2): 174–9.

47 Mieszczanska, H. et al. (2008). 'Gender-related differences in electrocardio graphic parameters and their association with cardiac events in patients after myocardial infarction'. In: *Am J Cardiol*, Jan 1; 101(1): 20–4.

48 Brenner, H. et al. (2010). 'Sex differences in performance of fecal occult blood testing'. In: *Am J Gastroenterol*, Nov; 105(11): 2457–64.

49 Glazerman, M. (2017). *Ook getest op vrouwen*. Veghel: Libris.

50 Westergaard, D. et al. (2019). 'Population-wide analysis of differences in disease progression patterns in men and women'. In: *Nat Commun*, Feb 8; 10(1): 666.

51 Tamargo, J. et al. (2017). 'Gender differences in the effects of cardiovascular drugs'. In: *Eur Heart J Cardiovasc Pharmacother*, July 1; 3(3): 163–82.

52 Pinn, V.W. (2013). 'Women's Health Research: Current State of the Art'. In: *Glob Adv Health Med*, Sept; 2(5): 8–10.

53 https://thoughtcatalog.com/lorenzo-jensen-iii/2015/06/14-real-physical-differences-between-men-and-women-besides-the-obvious/

54 Healy, B. (1991). 'The Yentl syndrome'. In: *N Engl J Med*, July 25; 325(4): 274–6.

55 Santin, A.P. et al. (2011). 'Role of estrogen in thyroid function and growth regulation'. In: *J Tyroid Res*: 875125.

56 Baumgartner, R.N. et al. (1999). 'Age-related changes in sex hormones affect the sex difference in serum leptin independently of changes in body fat'. In: *Metabolism*, Mar; 48(3): 378–84.

57 Shi, H. et al. (2009). 'Diet-induced obese mice are leptin insufficient after weight reduction'. In: *Obesity (Silver Spring)*, Sept; 17(9): 1702–9.

58 Jenks, M.Z. et al. (2017). 'Sex Steroid Hormones Regulate Leptin Transcript Accumulation and Protein Secretion in 3T3-L1 Cells'. In: *Sci Rep*, Aug 15; 7(1): 8232.

59 Vermeulen, A. et al. (1999). 'Testosterone, body composition and aging'. In: *J Endocrinol Invest*, 22(5 Suppl): 110–6.

60 Toss, F. et al. (2012). 'Body composition and mortality risk in later life'. In: *Age and Ageing*, Sept; 41(5): 677–81.

61 Baumgartner, R.N. et al. (1999). 'Predictors of skeletal muscle mass in elderly men and women'. In: *Mech Ageing Dev*, Mar 1; 107(2): 123–36.

62 Beld, A.W. van den, et al. (2018). 'The physiology of endocrine systems with ageing'. In: *Lancet Diabetes Endocrinol*, Aug; 6(8): 647–58.
63 Junnila, R.K. et al. (2013). 'The GH/IGH-1 axis in ageing and longevity'. In: *Nat Rev Endocrinol*, June; 9(6): 366–76.
64 Jones, C.M. et al. (2015). 'The Endocrinology of Ageing: A Mini-Review'. In: *Gerontology*, 61(4): 291–300.
65 Nunn, A.V.W. et al. (2009). 'Lifestyle-induced metabolic inflexibility and accelerated ageing syndrome: insulin resistance, friend or foe?'. In: *Nutr Metab (Lond)*, 6: 16.
66 Zaidi, M., et al. (2018). 'Actions of pituitary hormones beyond traditional targets'. In: *J Endocrinol*, June; 237(3): R83–R98.
67 Lamberts, S.W. et al. (1997). 'The endocrinology of aging'. In: *Science*, Oct 17; 278(5337): 419–24.
68 Liu, P. et al. (2017). 'Blocking FSH induces thermogenic adipose tissue and reduces body fat'. In: *Nature*, June 1; 546(7656): 107–112.
69 Pincus, S. (1996). 'Older males secrete luteinizing hormone and testosterone more irregularly, and jointly more asynchronously, than younger males'. In: *PNAS*, 93(24): 14100–5.
70 Verdile, G. et al. (2014). 'Associations between gonadotropins, testosterone and β amyloid in men at risk of Alzheimer's disease'. In: *Mol Psychiatry*, Jan; 19(1): 69–75.
71 Bhatta, S. et al. (2018). 'Luteinizing Hormone Involvement in Aging Female Cognition: Not All Is Estrogen Loss'. In: *Front Endocrinol (Lausanne)*, Sept 24; 9: 544.
72 Vinogradova, Y. et al. (2021). 'Use of menopausal hormone therapy and risk of dementia: nested case-control studies using QResearch and CPRD databases'. In: *BMJ*, Sep 29; 374: n2182.
73 Manson, J.E. et al. (2013). 'Menopausal hormone therapy and health outcomes during the intervention and extended poststopping phases of the Women's Health Initiative randomized trials'. In: *JAMA*, Oct 2; 310(13): 1353–68.
74 Bribiescas, R. (2010). *Evolutionary Endocrinology*. Cambridge University Press.
75 Charkoudian, N. et al. (2014). 'Reproductive hormone influences on thermoregulation in women'. In: *Compr Physiol*, Apr; 4(2): 793–804.
76 Bartke, A. (2008). 'Growth hormone and aging: a challenging controversy'. In: *Clin Interv Aging*, Dec; 3(4): 659–65.
77 https://en.wikipedia.org/wiki/Hara_hachi_bun_me
78 Marston, H.R. et al. (2021). 'A Commentary on Blue Zones®: A Critical Review of Age-Friendly Environments in the 21st Century and Beyond'. In: *Int J Environ Res Public Health*, Jan 19; 18(2): 837.
79 Willcox, B.J. et al. (2007). 'Caloric restriction, the traditional

Okinawan diet, and healthy aging: the diet of the world's longest-lived people and its potential impact on morbidity and life span'. In: *Ann N Y Acad Sci*, Oct; 1114(1): 434–55.

80  Karishma, K.K. et al. (2002). 'Dehydroepiandrosterone (DHEA) stimulates neurogenesis in the hippocampus of the rat, promotes survival of newly formed neurons and prevents corticosterone-induced suppression'. In: *Eur J Neurosci*, Aug; 16(3): 445–53.

81  Krokakai, K. et al. (2021). 'Correlation of age and sex with urine dehydroepiandrosterone sulfate level in healthy Tai volunteers'. In: *Pract Lab Med*, Mar; 24: e00204.

82  Sreekumaran Nair, K. et al. (2006). 'DHEA in elderly women and DHEA or testosterone in elderly men'. In: *N Engl J Med*, Oct 19; 355(16): 1647–59.

## Chapter 10 – Old Age

1  Billman, G.E. (2020). 'Homeostasis: The Underappreciated and Far Too Often Ignored Central Organizing Principle of Physiology'. In: *Front Physiol*, Mar 10; 11: 200.

2  Beld, A.W. van den, et al. (2018). 'The physiology of endocrine systems with ageing'. In: *Lancet Diabetes Endocrinol*, Aug; 6(8): 647–58.

3  Ennis, G.E. et al. (2017). 'Long-term cortisol measures predict Alzheimer disease risk'. In: *Neurology*, Jan 24; 88(4): 371–8.

4  Schoorlemmer, R.M.M. et al. (2009). 'Relationships between cortisol level, mortality and chronic diseases in older persons'. In: *Clin Endocrinol (Oxf)*, Dec; 71(6): 779–86.

5  Shin M.J. et al. (2018). 'Testosterone and Sarcopenia.' In: *World J Mens Health*, Sept; 36(3): 192–8.

6  Vajaranant, T.S. et al. (2012). 'Estrogen deficiency accelerates aging of the optic nerve'. In: *Menopause*, Aug; 19(8): 942–7.

7  Frisina, R.D. et al. (2021). 'Translational implications of the interactions between hormones and age-related hearing loss'. In: *Hear Res*, Mar 15; 402: 108093.

8  https://singularityhub.com/2018/05/03/is-the-secret-to-signifcantly-longer-life-hidden-in-our-cells/#sm.0001rlq28qruaef311rukgyhfsv5t

9  Huxley, A. (1939). *After Many a Summer*. London: Chatto & Windus.

10  Grey, A.D.N.J. de. (2015). 'Do we have genes that exist to hasten aging? New data, new arguments, but the answer is still no'. In: *Curr Aging Sci*, 8(1): 24–33.

11  https://en.wikipedia.org/wiki/Gilgamesh

12  https://en.wikipedia.org/wiki/Utnapishtim

13  https://www.nytimes.com/2012/12/02/magazine/can-a-jellyfish-unlock-the-secret-of-immortality.html?src=me&ref=general

14  Piraino, S. et al. (1996). 'Reversing the Life Cycle: Medusae Transforming into Polyps and Cell Transdifferentiation in Turritopsis nutricula (Cnidaria, Hydrozoa)'. In: *Biol Bull*, June; 190(3): 302–12.

15  Lisenkova, A.A. et al. (2017). 'Complete mitochondrial genome and evolutionary analysis of Turritopsis dohrnii, the "immortal" jellyfish with a reversible life-cycle'. In: *Mol Phylogenet Evol*, Feb; 107: 232–8.

16  https://opendata.cbs.nl/statline/#/cbs/nl/dataset/37360ned/table

17  https://www.ancient-origins.net/news-evolution-human-origins/life-expectancy-myth-and-why-many-ancient-humans-lived-long-077889

18  Nelson, P. et al. (2017). 'Intercellular competition and the inevitability of multicellular aging'. In: *Proc Natl Acad Sci USA*, Dec 5; 114(49): 12982–7.

19  Bliss, M. (2007). *Harvey Cushing: A Life in Surgery*. Oxford: Oxford University Press.

20  Descartes, R. (1664). *Traité de l'homme*. Paris: Charles Angot.

21  Zhang, Y. et al. (2017). 'Hypothalamic stem cells control ageing speed partly through exosomal miRNAs'. In: *Nature*, Aug 3; 548(7665): 52–7.

22  Spalding, K.L. et al. (2008). 'Dynamics of fat cell turnover in humans'. In: *Nature*, June 5; 453(7196): 783–7.

23  Zhang, G. et al. (2013). 'Hypothalamic programming of systemic ageing involving IKK-β, NF-KB and GnRH'. In: *Nature*, May 9; 497(7448): 211–16.

24  Mendelsohn, A.R. et al. (2017). 'Inflammation, Stem Cells, and the Aging Hypothalamus'. In: *Rejuvenation Res*, Aug; 20(4): 346–9.

25  Yoo, J. et al. (2017). 'Disability, Frailty and Depression in the community-dwelling older adults with Osteosarcopenia'. In: *BMC Geriatr*, Jan 5; 17(1): 7.

26  https://nl.wikipedia.org/wiki/Je_Echte_Leefijd

27  Jia, L. et al. (2017). 'Common methods of biological age estimation'. In: *Clin Interv Aging*, 12: 759–72.

28  Willcox, B.J. et al. (2007). 'Caloric restriction, the traditional Okinawan diet, and healthy aging: the diet of the world's longest-lived people and its potential impact on morbidity and life span'. In: *Ann N Y Acad Sci*, Oct; 1114: 434–55.

29  Orentreich, N. et al. (1984). 'Age changes and sex differences in serum dehydroepiandrosterone sulfate concentrations throughout adulthood'. In: *J Clin Endocrinol Metab*, Sept; 59(3): 551–5.

30  Sreekumaran Nair, K. et al. (2006). 'DHEA in elderly women and DHEA or testosterone in elderly men'. In: *N Engl J Med*, Oct 19; 355(16): 1647–59.

31  Ohayon, M.M. et al. (2004). 'Meta-analysis of quantitative sleep parameters from childhood to old age in healthy individuals:

developing normative sleep values across the human lifespan'. In: *Sleep*, Nov 1; 27(7): 1255–73.

32  Feng, R. et al (2016). 'Melanopsin retinal ganglion cell loss and circadian dysfunction in Alzheimer's disease'. In: *Mol Med Rep*, Apr; 13(4): 3397–400.

33  Scholtens, R.M. et al. (2016). 'Physiological melatonin levels in healthy older people: A systematic review'. In: *J Psychosom Res*, Jul; 86: 20–7.

34  Lockley, S.W. et al. (2007). 'Visual impairment and circadian rhythm disorders'. In: *Dialogues Clin Neurosci*; 9(3): 301–14.

35  Kocesvka, D. et al. (2021). 'Sleep characteristics across the lifespan in 1.1 million people from the Netherlands, United Kingdom and United States: a systematic review and meta-analysis'. In: *Nat Hum Behav*, Jan; 5(1): 113–22.

36  Klein, L. et al. (2017). 'Association between Sleep Patterns and Health in Families with Exceptional Longevity'. In: *Front Med (Lausanne)*, Dec 8; 4: 214.

37  Pierce, M. et al. (2019). 'Optimal Melatonin Dose in Older Adults: A Clinical Review of the Literature'. In: *Sr Care Pharm*, July 1; 34(7): 419–31.

38  Aarts, M.P.J. et al. (2018). 'Exploring the impact of natural light exposure on sleep of healthy older adults: A field study'. In: *Journal of Daylighting*, 5: 14–20.

39  Tähkämö, L. et al. (2019). 'Systematic review of light exposure impact on human circadian rhythm'. In: *Chronobiol Int*, Feb; 36(2): 151–70.

40  Buxton, O.M. et al. (1997). 'Acute and delayed effects of exercise on human melatonin secretion'. In: *J Biol Rhythms*, Dec; 12(6): 568–74.

41  Lanfranco, F. et al. (2003). 'Ageing, growth hormone and physical performance'. In: *J Endocrinol Invest*, Sept; 26(9): 861–72.

42  Rowe, J.W. et al. (1987). 'Human aging: usual and successful'. In: *Science*, July 10; 237(4811): 143–9.

43  Faulkner, J.A. et al. (2007). 'Age-related changes in the structure and function of skeletal muscles'. In: *Clin Exp Pharmacol Physiol*, Nov; 34(11): 1091–6.

44  Volaklis, K.A. et al. (2015). 'Muscular strength as a strong predictor of mortality: A narrative review'. In: *Eur J Intern Med*, June; 26(5): 303–10.

45  https://deadline.com/2021/01/worlds-oldest-marathon-runner-fauja-singh-biopic-indian-creative-trio-1234676075/

46  https://www.idfa.nl/nl/flm/c8d5cdde-bf25-488f-81ed-586422d5ffa8/autumn-gold46

47  Leon, J. et al. (2015). 'A combination of physical and cognitive exercise improves reaction time in persons 61–84 years old'. In: *J Aging Phys Act*, Jan; 23(1): 72–7.

# Notes

48 Forster, E.S. (1927). *The Works of Aristotle. Volume VII: Problemata*. (Translated into English under the editorship of W.D. Ross.) Oxford: Clarendon Press.

49 Martin, J. (2010). 'A functional ABCC11 allele is essential in the biochemical formation of human axillary odor'. In: *Journal of Investigative Dermatology*, 130(2): 529–40.

50 Honorat, M. et al. (2008). 'ABCC11 expression is regulated by estrogen in MCF7 cells, correlated with estrogen receptor alpha expression in postmenopausal breast tumors and overexpressed in tamoxifen-resistant breast cancer cells'. In: *Endocr Res Cancer*, 15(1): 125–38.

51 Lundstrom, J. et al. (2013). 'Maternal status regulates cortical responses to the body odor of newborns'. In: *Front Psychol*, 4: 597.

52 Fleming, A.S. et al. (1997). 'Cortisol, hedonics, and maternal responsiveness in human mothers'. In: *Horm Behav*, 32(2): 85–98.

53 Tang, W.H. (2013). 'Intestinal microbial metabolism of phosphatidylcholine and cardiovascular risk'. In: *NEJM*, 368: 1575–84.

54 Kootte, R.S. (2017). 'Improvement of Insulin Sensitivity after Lean Donor Feces in Metabolic Syndrome Is Driven by Baseline Intestinal Microbiota Composition'. In: *Cell Metabolism*, 26(4): 611–19.

55 Meijers, B.K.I. et al. (2010). 'p-Cresol and cardiovascular risk in mild-to-moderate kidney disease'. In: *Clin J Am Soci Neprhol*, 5(7): 1182–9.

56 Fluitman, K. et al. (2018). 'Potential of butyrate to influence food intake in mice and men'. In: *Gut*, 67(7): 1203–04.

57 Jalal, A.H. et al. (2018). 'Prospects and Challenges of Volatile Organic Compound Sensors in Human Healthcare'. *ACS Sens*, 27; 3(7): 1246–63.

58 Mitro, S. et al. (2012). 'The smell of age: perception and discrimination of body odors of different ages'. In: *PLoS One*, 7(5); e38110.

59 Kimura, K. (2016). 'Measurement of 2-nonenal and diacetyl emanating from human skin surface employing passive flux sampler-GCMS system'. In: *J Chromatogr B Analyt Biomed Life*, 1028: 181–5.

60 Yamazaki, S. et al; (2010). 'Odor Associated with Aging'. In: *Anti-Aging Medicine*, 7(6): 60–5.

61 McGee, H. (2020). *Nose Dive: A Field Guide to the World's Smells*. London: John Murray.

62 Lundstrom, J. (2010). 'Functional neuronal processing of human body odors'. In: *Vitam Horm*, 83: 1–23.

63 Mogilnicka, L. et al. (2020). 'Microbiota and Malodor – Etiology and Management'. In: *Int J Mol Sci*, Apr; 21(8): 2886.

64 Boesveldt, S. et al (2011). 'Gustatory and olfactory dysfunction

in older adults: a national probability study'. In: *Rhinology*, 49(3): 324–30.

65 Suzuki, K. et al. (2010). 'The role of gut hormones and the hypothalamus in appetite regulation'. In: *Endocr J*, 57(5): 359–72.

66 Castro, J.M. de (1993). 'Age-related changes in spontaneous food intake and hunger in humans'. In: *Appetite*, Dec; 21(3): 255–72.

67 Pelchat, M.L. et al. (2000). 'Dietary monotony and food cravings in young and elderly adults'. In: *Physiol Behav*, Jan; 68(3): 353–9.

68 MacIntosh, C.G. et al. (1999). 'Effects of age on concentrations of plasma cholecystokinin, glucagon-like peptide 1, and peptide YY and their relation to appetite and pyloric motility'. In: *Am J Clin Nutr*, 69: 999–1006.

69 Atalayer, D. et al. (2013). 'Anorexia of aging and gut hormones'. In: *Aging Dis*, Oct; 4(5): 264–75.

70 Amitani, M. et al. (2017). 'The Role of Ghrelin and Ghrelin Signaling in Aging'. In: *Int J Mol Sci*, July; 18(7): 1511.

71 Villa, A. et al. (2015). 'Diagnosis and management of xerostomia and hyposalivation'. In: *Ter Clin Risk Manag*, 11: 45–51.

72 Ohara, Y. et al. (2020). 'Association between anorexia and hyposalivation in community-dwelling older adults in Japan: a 6-year longitudinal study'. In: *BMC Geriatr*, 20: 504.

73 Fluitman K. et al. (2021). 'Poor Taste and Smell Are Associated with Poor Appetite, Macronutrient Intake, and Dietary Quality but Not with Undernutrition in Older Adults'. In: *J Nutr*, Mar 11; 151(3): 605–14.

74 Zemel, M.B. et al. (1988). 'Salt sensitivity and systemic hypertension in the elderly'. In: *Am J Cardiol*, 81: 7H–12H.

75 Park, S.Y. et al. (2018). 'Weight change in older adults and mortality: the Multiethnic Cohort Study'. In: *Int J Obes (Lond)*, Feb; 42(2): 205–12.

76 Veldhuis, J.D. (2008). 'Aging and hormones of the hypothalamo-pituitary axis: gonadotropic axis in men and somatotropic axes in men and women'. In: *Ageing Res Rev*, Jul; 7(3): 189–208.

77 Katsimpardi, L. et al. (2014). 'Vascular and neurogenic rejuvenation of the aging mouse brain by young systemic factors'. In: *Science*, May 9; 344(6184): 630–4.

78 https://unitybiotechnology.com

79 https://www.calicolabs.com

80 https://www.cnbc.com/2018/08/29/-jeff-bezos-is-backing-this-scientist-who-is-working-on-a-cure-for-aging.html

81 Scudellari, M. (2017). 'To stay young, kill zombie cells'. In: *Nature*, Oct 24; 550(7677): 448–50.

82 Xiao, Y.Z. et al. (2020). 'Reducing Hypothalamic Stem Cell Senescence Protects against Aging-Associated Physiological Decline'. In: *Cell Metab*, Mar 3; 31(3): 534–48.e5.

83 Baker, D.J. et al. (2011). 'Clearance of p16Ink4a-positive senescent

cells delays ageing-associated disorders'. In: *Nature*, Nov 2;
479(7372): 232–6.

84 Pajvani, U.B. et al. (2005). 'Fat apoptosis through targeted
activation of caspase 8: a new mouse model of inducible and
reversible lipoatrophy'. In: *Nat Med*, July; 11(7): 797–803.

85 https://www.ted.com/talks/
aubrey_de_grey_a_roadmap_to_end_aging/transcript

86 https://www.vpro.nl/programmas/tegenlicht/lees/bijlagen/2017-
2018/de-onsterfelijken/Pioniers-van-de-onsterfelijkheid-.html

87 Deursen, J.M. van (2014). 'The role of senescent cells in ageing'.
In: *Nature*, May 22; 509(7501): 439–46.

88 Skloot, R. (2010). *Het onsterfelijke leven van Henrietta Lacks*.
Amsterdam: Nieuw Amsterdam.

89 https://www.livescience.com/
henrietta-lacks-hela-cell-lawsuit-thermo-fisher

90 https://www.nobelprize.org/prizes/medicine/2009/
illustrated-information/

91 Shammas, M.A. (2011). 'Telomeres, lifestyle, cancer, and aging'.
In: *Curr Opin Clin Nutr Metab Care*, Jan; 14(1): 28–34.

92 Zglinicki, T. von, et al. (2005). 'Telomeres as biomarkers for
ageing and age-related diseases'. In: *Curr Mol Med*, Mar; 5(2):
197–203.

93 Epel, E.S. et al. (2004). 'Accelerated telomere shortening in
response to life stress'. In: *Proc Natl Acad Sci USA*, Dec 7; 101(49):
17312–5.

94 Movérare-Skrtic, S. et al. (2009). 'Serum insulin-like growth factor-
I concentration is associated with leukocyte telomere length in
a population-based cohort of elderly men'. In: *J Clin Endocrinol
Metab*, Dec; 94(12): 5078–84.

95 Verburgh, K. (2014). *The Food Hourglass: Stay Younger for Longer and
Lose Weight*. London: HarperCollins.

96 Johnson, R.J. et al. (2020). 'Fructose metabolism as a common
evolutionary pathway of survival associated with climate change,
food shortage and droughts'. In: *J Intern Med*, Mar; 287(3):
252–62.

97 Zheng, J. et al. (2017). 'Lower Doses of Fructose Extend Lifespan in
Caenorhabditis elegans'. In: *J Diet Suppl*, May 4; 14(3): 264–77.

98 Stephan, B.C.M. et al. (2010). 'Increased fructose intake as a risk
factor for dementia'. In: *J Gerontol A Biol Sci Med Sci*, Aug; 65(8):
809–14.

99 Leung, C.W. et al. (2014). 'Soda and cell aging: associations
between sugar-sweetened beverage consumption and leukocyte
telomere length in healthy adults from the National Health and
Nutrition Examination Surveys'. In: *Am J Public Health*, December;
104(12): 2425–31.

100 Sato, T. et al. (2019). 'Acute fructose intake suppresses

fasting-induced hepatic gluconeogenesis through the AKT-FoxO1 pathway'. In: *Biochem Biophys Rep*, Jul; 18: 100638.

101 Marissal-Arvy, N. et al. (2014). 'Effect of a high-fat–high-fructose diet, stress and cinnamon on central expression of genes related to immune system, hypothalamic-pituitary-adrenocortical axis function and cerebral plasticity in rats'. In: *Br J Nutr*, Apr 14; 111(7): 1190–201.

102 Dobson, A.J. et al. (2017). 'Nutritional Programming of Lifespan by FOXO Inhibition on Sugar-Rich Diets'. In: *Cell Rep*, Jan 10; 18(2): 299–306.

103 Boehm, A.M. et al. (2012). 'FOXO is a critical regulator of stem cell maintenance in immortal Hydra'. In: *Proc Natl Acad Sci USA*, Nov 27; 109(48): 19697–702.

104 Hsin, H. et al. (1999). 'Signals from the reproductive system regulate the lifespan of C. elegans'. In: *Nature*, May 27; 399(6734): 362–6.

105 Jasienska, G. et al. (2006). 'Daughters increase longevity of fathers, but daughters and sons equally reduce longevity of mothers'. In: *Am J Hum Biol*, May–June; 18(3): 422–5.

106 Jasienka, G. (2009). 'Reproduction and lifespan: Trade-offs, overall energy budgets, intergenerational costs, and costs neglected by research'. In: *Am J Hum Biol*, July–Aug; 21(4): 524–32.

107 Endendijk, J.J. et al. (2016). 'Gender-Differentiated Parenting Revisited: Meta-Analysis Reveals Very Few Differences in Parental Control of Boys and Girls'. In: *PLoS One*, July 14; 11(7): e0159193.

108 Arantes Oliveira, N. et al. (2003). 'Healthy animals with extreme longevity'. In: *Science*, Oct 24; 302(5645).

109 Chopik, W.J. (2018). 'Age Differences in Age Perceptions and Developmental Transitions'. In: *Front Pyschol*, 9: 67.

110 Lee, L.O. (2019). 'Optimism is associated with exceptional longevity in 2 epidemiologic cohorts of men and women'. In: *Proc Natl Acad Sci USA*, Sept 10; 116(37): 18357–362.

111 Li, S. et al. (2016). 'Association of Religious Service Attendance with Mortality Among Women'. In: *JAMA Intern Med*, June 1; 176(6): 777–85.

112 Seidman, S.N. et al. (2002). 'Low testosterone levels in elderly men with dysthymic disorder'. In: *Am J Psychiatry*, Mar; 159(3): 456–9.

113 Hogervorst, E. (2013). 'Effects of gonadal hormones on cognitive behaviour in elderly men and women'. In: *J Neuroendocrinol*, 25(11); 1182–95.

114 Zarrouf, F. et al. (2009). 'Testosterone and depression: systematic review and meta-analysis'. In: *J Psychiatr Pract*, Jul; 15(4): 289–305.

115 Yalamanchili, V. (2012). 'Treatment with hormone therapy and calcitriol did not affect depression in older postmenopausal women: no interaction with estrogen and vitamin D receptor genotype polymorphisms'. In: *Menopause*, June; 19(6): 697–703.

# Notes

116 Epel, E. (2009). 'Can meditation slow rate of cellular aging? Cognitive stress, mindfulness, and telomeres'. In: *Ann N Y Acad Sci*, Aug; 1172: 34–53.

## Epilogue

1 Ikegami, K. et al. (2019). 'Interconnection Between Circadian Clocks and Thyroid Function'. In: *Nat Rev Endocrinol*, Oct; 15(10): 590–600.

2 Wilson, L. et al. (2020). 'Dual-Hormone Closed-Loop System Using a Liquid Stable Glucagon Formulation Versus Insulin-Only Closed-Loop System Compared With a Predictive Low Glucose Suspend System: An Open-Label, Outpatient, Single-Center, Crossover, Randomized Controlled Trial'. In: *Diabetes Care*, Nov; 43(11): 2721–9.

3 Upton T. J., Zavala, E., Methlie, P. et al. (2023). 'High-resolution daily profiles of tissue adrenal steroids by portable automated collection'. In: *Science Translational Medicine*. 15(701): eadg8464.

4 Dutch medical oath (including Hippocratic Oath/Declaration of Geneva) directive, 2003.

# List of Hormones

adrenal gland hormone: see dehydroepiandrosterone (DHEA)

adrenaline

adrenocorticotropic hormone (ACTH)

aldosterone

antidiuretic hormone (ADH)

anti-Müllerian hormone (AMH)

bacteriocins (anti-inflammatory hormones)

cholecystokinin (CCK)

corticotropin-releasing hormone (CRH)

cortisol (stress hormone)

cuddle hormone: see oxytocin, prolactin

dehydroepiandrosterone (DHEA)

digestive hormone: see GLP-1, ptyalin

dopamine

EPO

follicle-stimulating hormone (FSH)

gastrin

ghrelin (hunger hormone)

GLP-1 (glucagon-like peptide 1)

glucagon

GnRH (gonadotropin-releasing hormone)

growth hormone (human growth hormone or HGH)

growth hormone-releasing peptides: see ghrelin

human chorionic gonadotropin (hCG)

IGF-1

inhibin B

insulin

leptin (satiety hormone)

LH (luteinising hormone)

melatonin (sleep hormone)

noradrenaline

oestradiol

oestrogen

oxytocin

parathyroid hormone (PTH)

pheromones

phytohormones

pregnancy hormone: see hCG

progesterone

prolactin

secretin

serotonin (mood hormone)

sex hormones

somatostatin

testosterone

thyroid hormone: see T4

T3 (triiodothyronine, active thyroid hormone)

T4 (thyroxin, thyroid hormone)

TRH

TSH

vasopressin: see ADH

# Index

Page references in *italics* indicate images.

333

# Index

# Index

# Index

# Index

Schubert, Franz: 'Erlkönig' 50–51
scoubidou craze 61
sebum 265
Second World War (1939–45) 65, 98, 115, 179, 190, 217, 252
secretin 7, 47, 332
*sedes stercoraria* ('excrement chair') 33–4
sella turcica 88
seminiferous tubule *20*
senolytics 271–2, 275
serotonin 14, 44, 83, 119, 120, 143, 153, 154, 158, 159, 235, 332
Sertoli cells 18
*Sesame Street* 82
Seveso disaster/TCDD 216
sexual attraction 14, *20*, 47, 83–5, 228
sexual preference 94–109
sexually dimorphic nucleus (SDN) 105–7, *106*
signalling molecules 7, 260–61
Simon, Eleazar ben 144–5
skin 14, 38, 44, 61, 67, *133*, 145, 158, 161, 162, 175, 187, 201, 232, 234–5, 258, 259, 265, 266, 267, 270
Skloot, Rebecca 272–3
sleep 13, 16, 37, 42, 46, 51
   biphasic 127
   children and 86, 89–91, 93
   gut and 160
   menopause and 202, 218
   obesity and 112, 126–8, 160
   old age and 252–3, *259*, 262–4, 274
   skin and 234
small intestine (duodenum) 119, *120*, 121, 123, 134, 143, 152, 159, 182
smell 65, 84, 85, 121, 142, 252, 264–7
Smith, Hayley 56
Socrates 175
Someren, Eus van 263
Sommer, Christian 255
soya 58, 59, 210
Spencer-Hall, Alicia: *Trans and Genderqueer Subjects in Medieval Hagiography* 96
sperm 14, 17–22, *20*, 23, 25, 26, 30, 31, 35, 60, 66, 71, 79, 169, 218
   crisis 19, 21–2
Starling, Ernest 7, 8
Statens Serum Institute, Copenhagen 101
stem cells 67, 254–5, 258–61, 270, 271, 273
stomach (gastrum) *12*, 13, 31, 40, 56, 83, 91, 118–24, *120*, *122*, 125, 126, 128, 129, 130, 131, 141–2, 143, 145, 146, 148, 152, 154, 155, 240, 272
stress 14, 16, 17, 24–5, 27, 48, *49*, 51–2, 76, 86, 92–3, 160, 261, 263, 266, 274, 275
   adrenal glands and 184–6, 188
   growth hormone and 92–3
   pain relief for physical 41–3
   pregnancy and 41–6
   sexual attraction and 83–4
   sexual identity and 107–8
   thyroid problems and 179–82, *183*
   weight and 110, 114, 126, 141
   yoga/breathing and 189–92
Struycken, Carel 87
Suez crisis (1956) 185–6
sugar 13, 14, 38, 42, 83, 84, 86, 91, 92, 119, 120, 121, *122*, 125–6, 134, 138, 140, 142, 152, *183*, 184, 192, 239, 274–6
suicide 170, 235–6
supplements 27, 34, 65, 67, 91, 101, 147, 169, 209, 210, 212, 226, 227, 248, 249, 250, 257
Swaab, Dick: *We Are Our Brains* 2, 41, 69, 102, 105, 106–7
Szostak, Jack 273

Talmud 144–5
taste 36, 65, 84, 139–40, 141–2, 147, 268–9
Tausk, Marius 136, 193
Taylor, Elizabeth 145
telomeres/telomerase 270, 273–5
testes/testicles 8, 9, *12*, 14, 18, *20*, 33–4, 37–8, 53, 62–8, 70, 71, 72, 95, 101, 131, 194, 195, 208, 225, 230
testosterone 8, 9, 10, 14
   ADAM/andropause and 224–5
   adrenal gland and 182, *183*, 184–5
   ageing and 226–8, 230, 231–2, 233, 234–5, 237, 247, 250, 253, 263–4
   contraceptive pill and 170–71
   obesity/hunger and 119, 137
   pregnancy/birth and 18, *20*, 22, *28*, 29, 32, 34, 36, 37, 44–5
   puberty and 53, 62, 63, 64, 65–71, 79–80, 84
   sexual identity and 95, 103, 104, 105, 107–8
   supplements 67, 227
   synthetic 187, 193–8
   thyroid and 181

343